'Cultural Life', Disability, Inclusion and Citizenship

Disability is a complex multidimensional social construct where the type of disability and the level of support of individuals needs to be considered within leisure provision. In a leisure context, people with a disability often face a multitude of constraints to participation. However, when leisure is possible, the benefits are substantial and worth pursuing. While other marginalised groups have received a great deal of attention across disciplines and in the field of leisure and recreation, disability has received comparatively less attention and generally in isolation to the leisure context. This book concentrates on "disability citizenship in leisure".

The chapters focus on examining the leisure lives of people with different types of disability by supporting their leisure endeavours through innovations in technology, service provision and the imagination. Each chapter has a different social setting, involves different groups of people with disability, and challenges conventional wisdom about what is possible when ability is seen, nurtured and, then, flourish as with the opportunities provided.

Rather than leisure being seen in isolation, the context of this book explores leisure as part of the everyday lives of people with disability whether that be part of promoting inclusive practices across understanding University campuses, invoking an innovative technology of Photovoice to allow people with intellectual disability to provide insight into their hopes and dreams of community living, maintaining mental health in refugees through innovative leadership programs, or examining how people with traumatic brain injury can regain autonomy through the arts. We situate the book in the context of further challenging researchers to think beyond disability as a context in their research and engage the person as a citizen for leisure opportunities, as opposed to a disability.

This book was published as a special issue of *Annals of Leisure Research*.

Simon Darcy is a Professor of Diversity Management at the Business School, University of Technology, Sydney. He is an interdisciplinary researcher with expertise in developing inclusive organisational approaches for diversity groups. Simon's work is characterised by implementing the outcomes of his research to change business, government and the not-for-profit sector's practice.

Jerome Singleton is a Professor of Leisure Studies; he is also cross-appointed with Faculty of Management, Nursing, Sociology and Social Anthropology at Dalhousie University. Jerry has published articles in a variety of publications such as the *Australian Journal of Occupational Science, Activities Adaptation and Aging, World Leisure Journal* and *Loisir/Leisure*. Jerome's research is based upon the intersection between Leisure and Aging and how they are interrelated to enhance a person's access to leisure across the life course.

'Cultural Life', Disability, Inclusion and Citizenship

Moving Beyond Leisure in Isolation

Edited by
Simon Darcy and Jerome Singleton

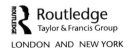

Routledge
Taylor & Francis Group

LONDON AND NEW YORK

First published 2015
by Routledge
2 Park Square, Milton Park, Abingdon, Oxon, OX14 4RN, UK

and by Routledge
711 Third Avenue, New York, NY 10017, USA

Routledge is an imprint of the Taylor & Francis Group, an informa business

British Library Cataloguing in Publication Data
A catalogue record for this book is available from the British Library

ISBN 13: 978-1-138-80992-5

Typeset in Times New Roman
by RefineCatch Limited, Bungay, Suffolk

Publisher's Note
The publisher accepts responsibility for any inconsistencies that may have
arisen during the conversion of this book from journal articles to book chapters,
namely the possible inclusion of journal terminology.

Disclaimer
Every effort has been made to contact copyright holders for their permission to
reprint material in this book. The publishers would be grateful to hear from any
copyright holder who is not here acknowledged and will undertake to rectify any
errors or omissions in future editions of this book.

Contents

Citation Information

The chapters in this book were originally published in *Annals of Leisure Research*, volume 16, issue 3 (October 2013). When citing this material, please use the original page numbering for each article, as follows:

Chapter 1
'Cultural life', disability, inclusion and citizenship: moving beyond leisure in isolation
Jerome Singleton and Simon Darcy
Annals of Leisure Research, volume 16, issue 3 (October 2013) pp. 183–192

Chapter 2
A framework for creating a campus culture of inclusion: a participatory action research approach
Jennifer Gillies and Sherry L. Dupuis
Annals of Leisure Research, volume 16, issue 3 (October 2013) pp. 193–211

Chapter 3
Using Photovoice to listen to adults with intellectual disabilities on being part of the community
Stuart J. Schleien, Lindsey Brake, Kimberly D. Miller and Ginger Walton
Annals of Leisure Research, volume 16, issue 3 (October 2013) pp. 212–229

Chapter 4
The relationship among motivational environment, autonomous self-regulation and personal variables in refugee youth: implications for mental health and youth leadership
Kiboum Kim, David M. Compton and Bryan McCormick
Annals of Leisure Research, volume 16, issue 3 (October 2013) pp. 230–251

Chapter 5
Enhancing communication between a person with TBI and a significant other through arts: pilot project
Hélène Carbonneau, Guylaine Le Dorze, France Joyal and Marie-Josée Plouffe
Annals of Leisure Research, volume 16, issue 3 (October 2013) pp. 252–268

Please direct any queries you may have about the citations to
clsuk.permissions@cengage.com

INTRODUCTION

'Cultural life', disability, inclusion and citizenship: moving beyond leisure in isolation

Jerome Singleton[a] and Simon Darcy[b]

[a]School of Health and Human Performance, Dalhousie University, Halifax, NS, Canada; [b]UTS Business School, University of Technology, Sydney, Australia

We reside within a global village, with approximately 10% of the world's population or 650 million people (including about 200 million children) living with some form of disability (United Nations 2011). This has been estimated to rise to 1.2 billion by 2050 (United Nations 2011). The World Health Organization and the United Nations have recognized that people with disability have a right to access services from all areas of citizenship. The purpose of this special issue of Annals of Leisure Research was to seek contributions examining the inclusion and citizenship of people with disability in 'cultural life', defined by the United Nation's (2006) Convention on the Rights of Persons with Disability (CRPWD) to include recreation, leisure, the arts, sport and tourism. In particular, the issue aimed to:

(1) clarify what the terms inclusion and citizenship mean in different cultures;
(2) place inclusion to and citizenship of 'cultural life' across discourses relating to economic, social and environmental contexts that affect people with disabilities participation; and
(3) discuss the terms inclusion and citizenship from the ideological frameworks of government, researchers, providers of service or disability advocacy groups.

Persons with differing levels of abilities

The first World Report on Disability (World Health Organization and World Bank 2011) shows that there are significant relationships between disability and ageing, relative quality of life and income, and relative health and country income status. The report goes on to document that 200 million people encounter significant difficulties in their daily life. They face barriers from the time they wake to the time they go to sleep again including: stigma and discrimination; lower levels of employment; lack of adequate health care and rehabilitation services; inaccessible transport; lack of access to the built environment; and communication/information. Table 1 (World Health Organization and World Bank 2011) presents the prevalence of disability across age,

Table 1. Prevalence of disability across high- and low-income countries (percent of population).

Population subgroup	Higher income countries	Lower income countries	All countries
Sex			
Male	9.1	13.8	12.0
Female	14.4	22.1	19.2
Age group			
18–49	6.4	10.4	8.9
50–59	15.9	23.4	20.6
≥ 60	29.5	43.4	38.1
Place of residence			
Urban	11.3	16.5	14.6
Rural	12.3	18.6	16.4
Wealth quintile			
Q1 (poorest)	17.6	22.4	20.7
Q2	13.2	19.7	17.4
Q3	11.6	18.3	15.9
Q4	8.8	16.2	13.6
Q5 (richest)	6.5	13.3	11.0
Total	11.8	18.0	15.6

Source: Adapted from World Health Organization and World Bank (2011, 28).

gender, place of residence and quartile of wealth based on showing the difference between high- and low-income nations.

These figures reinforce that disability is gendered, associated with ageing, more likely to be prevalent in rural areas, and is either related to income or more likely traps people in a poverty cycle. As others (e.g. Collins 2003) have observed, any one of these traits create significant social disadvantage. However, when two, three or four of these traits converge there is a magnification or a 'double whammy' effect that had been noted in groundbreaking studies on women with disability and leisure (Henderson and Bedini 1997; Henderson et al. 1995).

Overall, 16% of the global population experience some type of disability, a stark reminder that disability is a significant part of human diversity. Yet, people with disability are too often invisible in their own community, hidden from sight, restricted from participating, institutionalized and even those living in the community are sometimes unable to get outside their front door. The World Health Organization and the United Nations have recognized that people with disability have a right to access services from all areas of citizenship. The CRPWD can be thought of as a convention that elaborates the rights of people with disabilities and sets out a procedure for nation states to implement those rights. Some 154 nations have adopted the CRPWD. The CRPWD is based on eight principles:

- Respect for inherent dignity, individual autonomy including the freedom to make one's own choices, and independence of persons;
- Non-discrimination;
- Full and effective participation and inclusion in society;
- Respect for difference and acceptance of persons with disabilities as part of human diversity and humanity;
- Equality of opportunity;

- Accessibility;
- Equality between men and women;
- Respect for the evolving capacities of children with disabilities and respect for the rights of children with disabilities to preserve their identities.

The eight principles are a wonderful foundation for understanding the requirements for social participation and citizenship. People should be treated as individuals, in a dignified and equitable manner no matter what their ability or gender or age. They should be treated fairly before the law so as not to be discriminated against in their endeavours for full and active participation. Diversity should not only be accepted but celebrated as part of the wonder of humanity. To achieve social participation in the broader sense people require not only an equality of opportunity but an equitable opportunity that is founded on accessibility across disability types (e.g. mobility, vision, hearing, cognitive, etc.) and their support needs.

Article 30 of the CRPWD specifically recognizes 'cultural life' as an important part of any person's citizenship. As the CRPWD outlines, 'cultural life' is defined as including recreation, leisure, the arts, sport and tourism that can be regarded as the enriching part of people's lives where they strive to express themselves away from the everyday reality of their lifestyle situation and other constraints. Yet, people with disabilities participate less in all forms of social participation and specifically employment that define an individual's identity in most countries and provide the financial resources for freedom of choice during their leisure time (Barnes, Mercer, and Shakespeare 1999, 2010). Furthermore, a great deal of the lower levels of participation is due to discriminatory practices rather than a lack of desire to participate (Darcy and Taylor 2009; Genoe and Singleton 2009). Cultural life should be an area where people can freely express themselves, yet studies from all continents have clearly shown that this is not the case for people with disability.

As Stebbins (2007) and others (e.g. Darcy and Taylor 2009; Patterson 2007; DePauw and Gavron 2005; Smith et al. 2005) have argued, for some individuals and groups of people with disability, 'cultural life' plays a far more important role as they have been denied active citizenship in employment. Employment is a focus of citizenship, particularly in the neoliberal state, where denial of employment restricts income and, hence, choice in all other areas of life. A recent OECD (2010) report has shown that across nation states people with disability have much lower rates of employment than the non-disabled. For many, cultural life has become the 'serious' focus of their existence (Patterson 2007; Shaw and Dawson 2001; Stebbins 2000).

Providing a background for this special issue requires a brief examination of the history of the way that disability has been conceptualized in the twentieth century. The dominant model for understanding disability and social participation has come from medicalized approaches. These approaches to disability focus on the individual's impairment or as it is expressed, their health condition, disorder or disease. In short, medicalized approaches to disability view 'disability' as a deficit from the normal that requires interventional treatment to normalize the disabled body (Barnes, Mercer, and Shakespeare 2010). As shown in Figure 1, the World Health Organization's bio–psycho–social approach through the International Classification of Functioning (ICF) (World Health Organization 2001, 18) still has its foundations in medicalized approaches through focusing on the loss of function of a person before understanding their abilities.

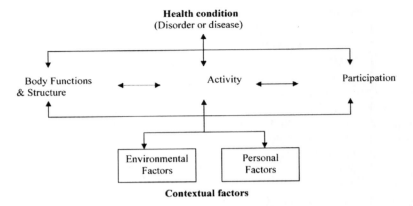

Figure 1. International classification of functioning.
Source: World Health Organization (2001).

The term 'activity' within Figure 1 is defined within the history and culture of each society based upon the environmental factors, personal factors, body function and structure of the person and the health conditions which influence the person's ability to participate in an activity. Central to the ICF is the intervention of medical and rehabilitation professionals to assist in maximizing capacity and performance based on body function and structures before examining the social and environmental context. The ICF model is currently being used in 161 nations to understand the abilities of their citizens. Individual's access to opportunities in cultural life sits at the intersection of the environment in which they reside, personal factors, body function and health conditions which may influence the person's abilities to engage in cultural activities within the community in which they reside. Yet, the foundation of this model still resides in a 'deficit' model of disability.

In contrast, the CRPWD takes a social model approach to understanding disability through the eight principles. This radically shifts the orientation away from 'normalizing' the body of the impaired individual by focusing on their lived experience, the disabling barriers that they face in the environment and the disabling attitudes of others towards them, and seeks a transformational outcome to create a more enabling environment (Barnes, Mercer, and Shakespeare 2010). The social approach to disability recognizes the importance of placing disability on the social, political, economic and cultural agendas. This is not to say that the individual's embodiment should not be considered within social model conceptualizations but that it should not be the starting point for inclusive practice. The importance of 'impairment effects' has been strongly advocated by feminist disability studies academics (e.g. Thomas 2004) within social model approaches. From a leisure studies perspective, this makes intuitive sense where understanding the individual as part of any response to members, clients or customers requires consideration of their level of ability in order to match their skills with the leisure challenges provided.

Connecting leisure research and disability studies

A lot has happened in the decade since Cara Aitchison (2003) drew our attention to the divide between disability research within leisure studies and leisure research within disability studies. In this very journal, a special issue (Darcy 2004) was dedicated to disability and leisure, which had its genesis at the 2003 Australian and New Zealand Association for Leisure Studies conference held in Sydney where a stream on the topic was held together with a series of performances by artists with disability, an integrated programme of accessible conference activities and inclusive educational practices. The special issue was dominated by papers examining innovative inclusive practice, and part of the issue was dedicated to a polemic examining the philosophical and theoretical divide between medical and social approaches to disability and leisure through which to establish a therapeutic recreation association in Australia (Fullagar and Darcy 2004; Stumbo, Martin, and Ogborne 2004).

While the debates between the dominant worldview and the challenge posed by social approaches continued, Cara Aitchison (2009) also identified how other theoretical and philosophical divides in the leisure studies traditions emanating from the sociology of work, geography of outdoor recreation and physical education have worked in combination to exclude an understanding of disability forged by disability studies, disability politics and disabled people themselves (Aitchison 2009). In recognizing this observation by Aitchison, the call for this issue has elicited some very important contributions to understanding disability from a social model perspective, through the voices of people with disabilities and others advocating enabling approaches that are underpinned by the principles of the CRPWD. We see the CRPWD as an opportunity to both reclaim the connection between leisure studies and disability studies, through the underlying social model approaches that give a voice to people with disabilities and their struggles to negotiate a dignified, equitable and independent leisure life no matter what their choice of activity, role or mode of engagement.

Participation is about choice across the continuum of participation in cultural life from segregated, inclusive, mainstream and universal approaches (DePauw and Gavron 2005; Smith et al. 2005). Figure 2 presents an understanding of these approaches in a sporting context, where the goal is to provide people with disability choice to participate in sport in the way that they want to, with whom they want to participate and in the way they wish to participate. The Australian Sports Commission's Disability Sport Unit developed the Inclusion Spectrum For Disability Sport (Australian Sports Commission Disability Sport Unit 2010), where the spectrum is used to provide an understanding of type of engagement and level of modification that may be required for participation of people with disability. A person may choose to participate in any part of the spectrum, depending on their ability, the sport in which they are participating, the opportunities within their local environment and their personal preferences. As Darcy et al. (2011) go on to describe, the inclusion spectrum covers:

- No modifications: for example, an athlete with an intellectual disability may train and compete with athletes without intellectual disability at a local swimming club.
- Minor modifications: for example, a vision-impaired tenpin bowler using a rail to steady themself.
- Major modifications: for example, a seated shot-putter competing under separate rules using modified equipment against other athletes with disability in an integrated track and field competition.

- Primarily for people with disability: for example, athletes with disability and their able-bodied peers combine to form teams for the purpose of developing a wheelchair basketball competition.
- Only for people with disability: for example, goalball players participating in a competition exclusively for people with vision impairments.
- Non-playing role: people with disability can be officials, coaches, club presidents, volunteers, spectators (Figure 2).

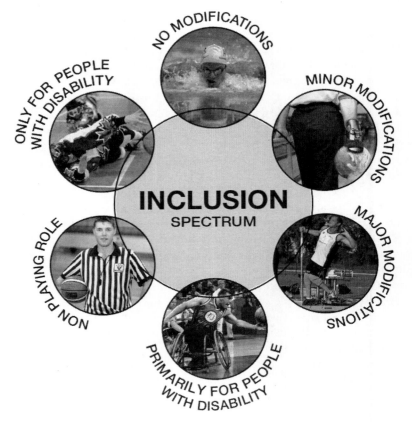

Figure 2. Inclusion spectrum.
Source: Australian Sports Commission Disability Sport Unit (2010).

The type of approach advocated by the Australian Sports Commission has been operationalized in other parts of the world including London. The London 2012 Olympic and Paralympic Games were seen as an opportunity for the UK to challenge their citizen's attitudes and behaviours towards the way that they think about people with disability. In doing so, the Games committee wanted to increase the integration of people with disability across all involvements with the Games including participation as elite athletes, involvement in the cultural Olympiad, an equality of experience as spectators, involvement in volunteer programmes and as employees of the organization. Quite simply they saw the Games as a watershed moment to leverage a social legacy of wider community involvement for people with disability that could be beneficial to all (Volunteering England 2011). The London

Games spoke of diversity, equity and inclusion as founding pillars of a more just society. Let's hope the UK government can continue such a visionary idea beyond the Games when the international spotlight and media attention is no longer prevalent. The Sydney 2000 Olympic and Paralympic Games' experience suggests that once the relief of staging a 'successful' Games has subsided, the budgetary reality sets in, the political will wanes and the spotlight on disability dissipates over the coming years (Cashman and Darcy 2008; Darcy 2003). Yet, it is with this hope set by the London experience that we present this special issue of the Annals of Leisure Research and papers that explore the underlying principles of the CRPWD across disability type, people with different support needs and in very different leisure contexts.

Articles in special issue

The articles within this special issue provide insights into inclusion and citizenship of people with disability in their cultural life through the lens of the environment that the person resides in (university, city, rehabilitation facility or country). Citizens of any nation who have varying levels of abilities are engaged in activities such as education, work and leisure (Stumbo and Singleton 2007; Genoe and Singleton 2009). Children and families of children with a disability are confronted with a variety of issues from social supports to access to appropriate learning environments that would enable the children and family members to achieve their optimal level of ability. Access and use of recreation opportunities for the person with various levels of abilities and family members have been examined within the literature (Schleien and Wehman 1984; Schleien, Ray, and Green 1997; Mactavish and Schleien 2000). The acquisitions of a leisure repertoire for a citizen with various levels of abilities will enable the citizen to gain access to other culture experiences as he or she enters different social groups (Patterson 2000; Pegg and Darcy 2007; Schleien, Miller, and Shea 2009; Schleien, Germ, and McAvoy 1996; Schleien, Green, and Stone 1999).

What can universities do to include citizens with various abilities in their community? Gillies and Dupuis provide insights into how participatory action research assists in making a university accessible and an inclusive community for all individuals who work, study, live or visit the campus. They interviewed 23 stakeholders (faculty members, university administrators and students) which provided six guiding principles: (1) access for all, (2) value the diversity and uniqueness of all, (3) value interdependence and social responsibility, (4) value diverse knowledge bases, voices and perspectives, (5) value the power of learning and education as tools for growth and change and (6) value the whole person; and three characteristics for creating a campus culture of inclusion: (1) an Interconnected Campus Community, (2) a Supportive and Enabling Campus Community and (3) an Informed Campus Community.

Communities have an impact on a person's ability to access and use resources. How a person views their community will be influenced by their stage of life course, gender, culture and level of abilities. Schleien, Brake, Miller, & Walton demonstrate how Photovoice provides insights into the interests, hopes and dreams of persons with intellectual or developmental disabilities who reside in the community. Seven individuals participated in this qualitative study, where the authors found out that 'community membership and desire for independence' emerged as the overriding themes. These themes of belonging and independence are universal yet denied to people with intellectual disability in almost every facet of their lives. Photovoice provides an insight into their world, through their eyes and provides evidence through an innovative approach that gives us a much better understanding of a group that wants to be visible.

We reside in a global community where each year approximately 20 million citizens move from developing nations to developed nations (Bloom and Canning 2006). This migration of people has an impact on the citizens relocating as well as the citizens that they come in contact with in their new communities. North America is becoming more diverse as the result of migration. The term 'leisure' needs to be reconsidered as the result of the influence of the various cultures on the community they have migrated to (Iwaski et al. 2007). The question arises, how does the migration impact on the youth who have moved from one culture to a North American culture? Kim, Compton & McCormick's study provides insights into how leisure assists in making the transition of refugee youth in relation to self-regulation. Youth from refugee backgrounds have much higher levels of mental health-related issues due to issues with acculturation (Okigbo, Reierson, and Stowman 2009). This timely study provides a background of these issues and how an innovative leadership programme has been able to assist those participating in the acculturation process. Eighteen refugee youth participated in the qualitative study. The authors found that gender, experience and the autonomy of a supportive environment were predictors of self-regulation. The leadership programme is one example of the type of interventions that can assist in the transition from developing nations to developed nations, provide a focus for individuals in their leisure time and lead to lower levels of mental health issues during this turbulent period in the refugees' lives.

Individuals who have traumatic brain injury (TBI) go through social, physical and cognitive transitions due to their new abilities. These transitions affect the person as well as their family members. What role can a leisure experience such as art play in coping with loss of autonomy and connecting with family? Carbonneau, Le Dorze, Joyal, & Plouffe provide a lens into how involvement in the arts could assist in the loss of autonomy and how it enhances social relations with caregivers. The results of the study found that the dyads perceptions of social engagement were altered as a result of their experience in the arts programme.

Citizenship is how individuals gain access to opportunities based upon what resources are available in a person's community. The articles in this special issue provide insights into how citizens (new immigrants with mental health issues, persons with developmental abilities, persons with a disability, persons who have acquired a condition such as a TBI) were provided access to leisure opportunities. The diversity of the lens of the researchers and people with disability in this special issue reflect an understanding of the issues that confront individuals and organizations being inclusive of 'citizens' rather than focusing upon the deficits of the individuals.

Disability is a continually evolving area of scholarship where what was once considered cutting edge is now considered standard and mainstream. While there has been a great focus on people with mobility disability, this special issue has presented some fascinating studies involving people with intellectual disability, traumatically acquired brain injury and mental health. We can only imagine what the international focus of the CRPWD will create, inspire and how it will provide the impetus for people with disability to create the leisure lives that they desire in the future.

We, the guest editors hope you get as much enjoyment reading the contributions as we did assisting the authors to make the contributions. We also wanted to thank all the reviewers who contributed to shaping the articles as it is their volunteered time that journals like Annals of Leisure Research are so heavily reliant on. Lastly, to other authors who have an interest in this area we implore you to come forward with your contributions and add to this very important body of knowledge.

References

Aitchison, C. 2003. "From Leisure and Disability to Disability Leisure: Developing Data, Definitions and Discourses." *Disability & Society* 18 (7): 955–969. doi:10.1080/09687590 32000127353

Aitchison, C. 2009. "Exclusive Discourses: Leisure Studies and Disability." *Leisure Studies* 28 (4): 375–386. doi:10.1080/02614360903125096

Australian Sports Commission Disability Sport Unit. 2010. *Australian Inclusion Spectrum.* Canberra: Australian Sports Commission and Standing Committee on Recreation and Sport.

Barnes, C., G. Mercer, and T. Shakespeare. 1999. "Culture, Leisure and the Media." In *Exploring Disability: A Sociological Introduction*, edited by C. Barnes, G. Mercer, and T. Shakespeare, 182–210. Malden, MA: Polity Press.

Barnes, C., G. Mercer, and T. Shakespeare. 2010. *Exploring Disability: A Sociological Introduction.* 2nd ed. Malden, MA: Polity Press.

Bloom, D. E., and D. Canning. 2006. *Global Demography: Fact, Force and Future.* The WDA-HSG Discussion Paper Series on Demographic Issues, No. 2006/1, World Demographic Association, Accessed February 20, 2007. http://www.wdassociation.org/ulfs/documents/WDA-HSG-DP2006-1_Bloom_Canning.pdf

Cashman, R., and S. Darcy, eds. 2008. *Benchmark Games: The Sydney 2000 Paralympic Games.* Petersham, NSW: Walla Walla Press in Conjunction with the Australian Centre for Olympic Studies.

Collins, M. F. 2003. "Social Exclusion from Sport and Leisure." In *Sport and Society: A Student Introduction*, edited by Barry Houlihan. 77–105. London: Sage.

Darcy, S. 2003. "The Politics of Disability and Access: The Sydney 2000 Games Experience." *Disability & Society* 18 (6): 737–757. doi:10.1080/0968759032000119497

Darcy, S. 2004. "Guest Editors' Introduction." *Annals of Leisure Research* 7 (2): vi–viii. doi:10.1080/11745398.2004.10600942

Darcy, S., and T. Taylor. 2009. "Disability Citizenship: An Australian Human Rights Analysis of the Cultural Industries." *Leisure Studies* 28 (4): 419–441. doi:10.1080/026143609030 71753

Darcy, S., T. Taylor, A. Murphy, and D. Lock. 2011. *Getting Involved in Sport: The Participation and Non-Participation of People with Disability in Sport and Active Recreation.* Canberra: Australian Sport Commission.

DePauw, K. P., and S. J. Gavron. 2005. *Disability and Sport.* 8th ed. Champaign, IL: Human Kinetics.

Fullagar, S., and S. Darcy. 2004. "Critical Points against an Australasian Therapeutic Recreation Association: Towards Community Leisure through Enabling Justice." *Annals of Leisure Research* 7 (2): 95–103. doi:10.1080/11745398.2004.10600944

Genoe, R., and J. F. Singleton. 2009 "World Demographics and Their Implications for Therapeutic Recreation." In *Professional issues in therapeutic recreation on competence and outcomes*, edited by N. J. Stumbo, 31–42. Champaign, IL: Sagamore.

Henderson, K. A., and L. A. Bedini. 1997. "Women, Leisure, and 'double whammies': Empowerment and Constraint." *Journal of Leisurability* 24 (1): 36–46.

Henderson, K., L. Bedini, L. Hecht, and R. Schuler. 1995. "Women with Physical Disabilities and the Negotiation of Leisure Constraints." *Leisure Studies* 14 (1): 17–31. doi:10.1080/02614369500390021

Iwasaki, Y., H. Nishino, T. Onda, and C. Bowling. 2007. "Research Reflections Leisure Research in a Global World: Time to Reverse the Western Domination in Leisure Research?" *Leisure Sciences* 29 (1): 113–117. doi:10.1080/01490400600983453

OECD. 2010. *Sickness, Disability and Work: Breaking the Barriers: A Synthesis of Findings across OECD Countries.* Geneva: OECD.

Okigbo, C., J. Reierson, and S. Stowman. 2009. "Leveraging Acculturation through Action Research a Case Study of Refugee and Immigrant Women in the United States. *Action Research* 7 (2): 127–142. doi:10.1177/1476750309103267

Patterson, I. 2000. "Developing a Meaningful Identity for People with Disabilities through Serious Leisure Activities." *World Leisure Journal* 42 (2): 41–51. doi:10.1080/04419057. 2000.9674185

Patterson, I. 2007. "Changes in the Provision of Leisure Services for People with Disabilities in Australia." *Therapeutic Recreation Journal* 41 (2): 108–118.

Pegg, S., and S. Darcy. 2007. "Sailing on Troubled Waters: Diversional Therapy in Australia." *Therapeutic Recreation Journal* 41 (2): 132–140.

Schleien, S. J., P. A. Germ, and L. McAvoy. 1996. "Inclusive Community Leisure Services: Recommended Professional Practices and Barriers Encountered." *Therapeutic Recreation Journal* 30 (4): 260–273.

Schleien, S., F. Green, and C. Stone. 1999. "Making Friends within Inclusive Community Recreation Programs." *Journal of Leisurability* 26 (3): 33–43.

Schleien, S. J., K. D. Miller, and M. Shea. 2009. "Search for Best Practices in Inclusive Recreation: Preliminary Findings." *Journal of Park & Recreation Administration* 27 (1): 17–34.

Schleien, S. J., M. T. Ray, and F. P. Green. 1997. *Community Recreation and People with Disabilities: Strategies for Inclusion*. 2nd ed. Baltimore: Paul Brookes.

Schleien, S. J., and P. Wehman. 1984. *Leisure Programs for Handicapped Persons*. Baltimore, MD: University Park Press.

Shaw, S. M., and D. Dawson. 2001. "Purposive Leisure: Examining Parental Discourses on Family Activities." *Leisure Sciences* 23 (4): 217–231. doi:10.1080/01490400152809098

Smith, R., D. R. Austin, D. W. Kennedy, Y. Lee, and P. Hutchison. 2005. *Inclusive and Special Recreation: Opportunities for Persons with Disabilities*. 5th ed. New York: McGraw Hill.

Stebbins, R. A. 2000. "Serious Leisure for People with Disabilities." In *Leisure Education, Community Development and Populations with Special Needs*, edited by A. Sivan and H. Ruskin, 101–108. Wallingford: CABI.

Stebbins, R. A. 2007. *Serious Leisure: A Perspective for Our Time*. New Brunswick, NJ: Transaction Pub.

Stumbo, N. J., L. D. Martin, and V. Ogborne. 2004. "Collective Voices, Shared Wisdom: On the Need for a Professional Association to Represent Therapeutic Recreation in Australia." *Annals of Leisure Research* 7 (2): 85–94. doi:10.1080/11745398.2004.10600943

Stumbo, N., and J. Singleton. 2007. "Introduction to Special Issue Globalization of Therapeutic Recreation." *Therapeutic Recreation Journal* 41 (2): 106–107.

Thomas, C. 2004. "Disability and Impairment." In *Disabling Barriers-Enabling Environments*, edited by J. Swain, S. French, C. Barnes, and C. Thomas, 21–28. London: SAGE.

United Nations. (2006). *Convention on the Rights of Persons with Disabilities*. New York Nations General Assembly A/61/611. http://www.un.org/esa/socdev/enable/rights/convtexte. htm: United.

United Nations. (2011). *Enable*. Accessed June 2, 2011. http://www.un.org/disabilities/

Volunteering England. (2011). *Volunteering England Statement–London 2012 Olympic and Paralympic Games Legacy*. Volunteering England. Accessed November 18, 2011. http://www.volunteering.org.uk/WhatWeDo/Policy/whatwearesaying/Volunteering+England+Statement+-+London+2012+Olympic+and+Paralympic+Games+legacy

World Health Organization. (2001). *International Classification of Functioning, Disability and Health*. Geneva: World Health Organization.

World Health Organization and World Bank. (2011). *World Report on Disability*. http://www.who.int/disabilities/world_report/2011/report/en/index.html

A framework for creating a campus culture of inclusion: a participatory action research approach

Jennifer Gillies[a] and Sherry L. Dupuis[b]

[a]*Alzheimer Societies of Kitchener-Waterloo, Cambridge, and Guelph-Wellington, Kitchener, Canada;* [b]*Department of Recreation and Leisure Studies, University of Waterloo, Waterloo, Canada*

This study used a participatory action research (PAR) approach to unite key partners from the University of Guelph community in order to examine issues around accessibility and inclusion of students with disabilities in campus life. The goal was to develop a planning framework to assist universities in creating accessible and inclusive campus communities that supports not only students with disabilities, but all individuals who study, live, work or visit the campus. Interviews were conducted with 23 University of Guelph stakeholders, including students with and without disabilities, staff and faculty members, and senior administrators. What emerged was a framework for Creating a Campus Culture of Inclusion. The framework centres around six guiding principles and three fundamental characteristics that a campus culture of inclusion must possess. Process pieces are included in the framework which help fuel and sustain the culture over time.

Background

Approximately 650 million individuals worldwide are living with a disability and, as a result, experience physical, social, economic and systemic barriers that prevent them from gaining experiences and accessing opportunities provided to the mainstream population (United Nations 2006). There have been vast inconsistencies in the legislations protecting the rights of persons with disabilities across the world. In an effort to rectify this, the United Nations implemented a convention on the rights of persons with disabilities to 'promote, protect, and ensure the full and equal enjoyment of all human rights by persons with disabilities' (United Nations 2006, 1). Countries that ratify the convention will be obligated to take measures to promote the human rights of persons with disabilities, including legislations and policies that promote accessibility within various facets of life, including education (United Nations 2006).

The global movement towards promoting and protecting the rights of persons with disabilities has influenced the infrastructure, and administration, of post-secondary institutions. Globally, universities are actively creating accessible spaces, policies, and practices to enable persons with disabilities to access, and reap the benefits of, a post-secondary education. In 2012, for example, Israel allocated 90 million dollars to enhance the accessibility of university campuses by 2014 to adhere to 'equal opportunity' laws for persons with disabilities passed in 2005 (Dattel 2012). Until now, universities were either completely inaccessible, or only partially accessible, to persons with physical or sensory disabilities (Dattel 2012). In 2013, South Africa's Deputy Minister of the Department of Women, Children and People with Disabilities visited South African universities to assess their accessibility and treatment of students with disabilities. The Minister urged universities to open disability rights offices to promote and protect the rights of students and employees with disabilities and ensure compliance with universal disability access principles (South African Government Information 2013). Similar movements towards enhancing access to universities have been seen around the world. A cursory review of university websites across North America, the UK and beyond will often reveal the existence of offices and services that support the rights and inclusion of students with disabilities.

In Canada, provincial and federal anti-discrimination legislation has resulted in an increase of students with disabilities attending Canadian universities (Department of Justice Canada 1982; Duquette 2000; Legislative Assembly of Ontario 2004). Although their presence on campus is increasing, Canadian students with disabilities continue to be marginalized within universities, mainly because a framework for inclusion has not been firmly established (Merchant and Gajar 1997; Promis, Erevelles, and Matthews 2001). Most Canadian universities support students with disabilities by providing on-campus support services, often through an office for students with disabilities, which address structural and attitudinal barriers on campus. Although support services catering to students' needs are beneficial, it is problematic when universities solely rely on these services to ensure students are included and accommodated within various elements of campus life. This traditional framework places accommodation and inclusion as afterthoughts, post hoc solutions to 'problems' associated with disability. Although a campus office for students with disabilities may serve to support specific student concerns and accommodations, diversity and inclusion within the broader university environment must be viewed as an integral part of the campus culture and structure.

Another concern with on-campus support services for persons with disabilities is that they typically focus on the academic side of life, while other facets of university life are not fully addressed (Promis, Erevelles, and Matthews 2001). These social areas of university life should not be considered trivial (Promis, Erevelles, and Matthews 2001), since research clearly indicates that recreation and athletic opportunities have many benefits and can enhance a person's experiences and quality of life at university (Ashton-Shaeffer et al. 2001; Blinde and McLung 1997; Blinde and Taub 1999; Promis, Erevelles, and Matthews 2001). University students, in particular, benefit from such activities because they assist in academic stress relief, foster a sense of community, help develop leadership skills and foster teamwork and team building (Promis, Erevelles, and Matthews 2001). Despite these known benefits, students with disabilities are often excluded from campus recreation and athletics, which includes informal and formal sports (e.g., intramural and varsity sports) and recreation opportunities (e.g., fitness classes), because such activities are not fully accessible, inclusive or designed to meet their needs or preferences (Ashton-Shaeffer et al. 2001). Moreover, many persons with disabilities have been raised in a culture that has not fostered their athletic and recreation aspirations. People with disabilities often lack sporting programs and opportunities within their community and face stigmatization and prejudices when participating. Sports facilities and recreation environments are often inaccessible, and coaching and training opportunities are often not a priority for sports catering to persons with disabilities (Ashton Shaeffer et al. 2001; DePauw 1997; DePauw and Gavron 2005; Promis, Erevelles, and Matthews 2001).

Research has not fully explored the role of Canadian universities in providing athletic and campus recreational opportunities for students with disabilities. Literature regarding campus athletics has typically focused on American universities and has mainly explored the effects of campus athletics on stigma management (Taub, Blinde, and Greer 1999) and reported the benefits and barriers to campus athletics (Ashton-Shaeffer et al. 2001; Blinde and McLung 1997; Blinde and Taub 1999; Promis, Erevelles, and Matthews 2001). Benefits cited in this literature include the ability of persons with disabilities to experience their body in various physical ways, enhanced perceptions of physical attributes and physical capabilities, and an enhancement of confidence (Promis, Erevelles, and Matthews 2001; Ashton-Shaeffer et al. 2001). Further, opportunities for recreation and athletics between those with and without disabilities help to break down stereotypes while increasing positive perceptions of persons with disabilities by their non-disabled peers (Ashton-Shaeffer et al. 2001; Blinde and Taub 1999; Blinde and McLung 1997).

In an earlier study conducted by the first author, the official websites of seventeen accredited Ontario Universities were examined to determine the availability of on-campus athletic opportunities for students with disabilities and the extent to which these opportunities were promoted (Gillies 2005). Findings revealed a general lack of advertised athletic opportunities for university students with disabilities. Of the seventeen universities, only five promoted disability awareness campaigns where sporting events, such as wheelchair sports, were used to raise disability awareness. Six universities promoted the incorporation of athletes with disabilities (such as Paralympians) in varsity training and/or teams. Only five universities featured adapted athletic opportunities for students with disabilities, such as intramural wheelchair basketball or able-swim. A lack of opportunities was evident in cases relating to non-athletically elite students. It was positive that nearly every university promoted some commitment towards achieving physically accessible athletic complexes, including gymnasiums, arenas or pools. That this type of accommodation was common may be because Ontario universities are required under provincial legislation to create and post accessibility plans which aim to attain physically accessible buildings on campus (Ontario Ministry of Community and Social Services 2008). However, a lack of a minimal accessibility standard within Canadian universities has resulted in post-secondary institutions interpreting their responsibility with regard to accessibility and inclusion related to the built environment. What is problematic is that without strict and broader accessibility and inclusion guidelines, universities may not have the information or support necessary to be proactive (or even reactive) in striving to make their environments accessible and equitable to all of the citizens who study, work, live and visit the university.

This study began with an interest in exploring issues of accessibility, inclusion and opportunities for students with disabilities as they pertain to participation in campus recreation and athletics. We chose a participatory action research (PAR) approach as a means to unite key university and community stakeholders in order to examine issues around accessibility and inclusion of students with disabilities in campus life. We began by exploring how the planning, development and implementation of campus recreation and athletics programs, services, policies and/or practices could enhance the well-being of community members, particularly students with disabilities. As we progressed with the research, it became clear that what we were uncovering and developing captured far more than involvement in recreation, leisure and sport on university campuses; we were getting at key aspects of supporting life more broadly, not only for persons with disabilities but for all those engaged in university campuses. We turned our attention to developing a planning framework to support universities in creating an accessible and inclusive campus community that supports not only students with disabilities, but all individuals who study, live, work or visit the campus. Thus, our approach extended beyond the exploration of the role of academic supports for persons with disabilities, as well as a focus on the benefits of recreation and athletics, towards a more holistic approach to enhancing all aspects of campus life, including extra-curricular engagement.

The study was guided by critical disability theory and the concept of embodiment. Critical disability theory is built upon the assertion that 'disability is not fundamentally a question of medicine or health, nor is it just an issue of sensitivity and compassion; rather, it is a question of politics and power(lessness), power over, and power to' (Devlin and Pothier 2006, 2). Critical disability theory extends beyond the individual pathology of disability (the biomedical model) towards a human rights approach that argues for equal access to aspects of social life (Gillies 2012; Oliver 1993) as well as 'key sites of power and privilege' (Hughes and Paterson 1997, 325). This perspective challenges the oppression that arises from restricting economic and social benefits to persons with disabilities (Gillies 2012; Oliver 1993; Rioux and Frazee 1999; Rioux and Prince 2002). We further acknowledge that while disability is socially and politically constructed, it is also an embodied personal experience (Hughes and Paterson 1997; Turner 2001; Williams 2008; Zola 1993). Disability involves a complex interplay between social oppression and human affliction (Hughes and Paterson 1997); thus, the experience of disability and how disability is embodied cannot be omitted.

Method

A PAR team was formed in 2008 with the University of Guelph and community members who play a role in the administration, provision and utilization of campus supports for persons with disabilities and extra-curricular engagement. The University of Guelph was selected as the study site because they were identified as one of the few Canadian Universities that demonstrated a commitment to increasing equity in their recreation programmes (Gillies 2005). The research team included two staff members and one student from the University of Guelph, two university alumni and the primary author who was a doctoral student at the time. Four of the research team members are living with a disability. The team collaboratively designed the research project, provided insights throughout the process, was involved in all major decision-making and reviewed a synthesized report of the findings. The project was completed in the Fall of 2010.

The research team recruited participants through purposeful and snowball sampling. Information letters outlining the study and inviting persons to participate were emailed to students registered with the Centre for Students with Disabilities (CSD) on behalf of the research team using the CSD student database. However, only two students were recruited using this approach. Recruitment posters were also displayed around the campus (e.g., CSD offices and athletic change rooms and facilities) which prompted several students without disabilities to participate. The remaining students, both with and without disabilities, volunteered to participate after learning more about the project from their CSD advisor, on-campus employer (Department of Athletics) or class mates who were involved in the study. A special effort was made to include students with mental health issues in the study. As such, a CSD advisor talked to her students with mental health issues about the study; however, none contacted the researcher to participate. We worked with the CSD advisor to explore other ways of including their perspective beyond the traditional interview approach, but after a continued lack of response from these students, we decided it was important to respect their privacy and discontinue additional recruitment strategies. As the study unfolded, members of the PAR team identified other key informants whose perspective would be an asset to the study (e.g., staff members with disabilities, members of the University's Accessibility for Persons with Disabilities Advisory Committee and senior level administrators) and invited them to participate via email. In order to protect anonymity, persons interested in participating in the study contacted the lead author (who was doing her degree at another southwestern Ontario university in Canada) to participate.

Throughout the process, active interviews were conducted with 18 participants and 5 research team members, amounting to 23 interviews in total. Specifically, the lead author met individually with: (1) six students with varying disabilities including cerebral palsy, acquired brain injury, visual impairments and fibromyalgia, (2) two alumni with disabilities including muscle-skeletal disabilities and a visual impairment; (3) four staff members from the CSD who specialize in areas of mental health, learning disabilities and physical and temporary disabilities; (4) six students without disabilities, one of which was a Resident Advisor and five who were part-time staff members with the Department of Athletics; (5) three staff members in management positions; (6) one faculty member who Chairs the University's Accessibility for Persons with Disabilities Advisory Committee and (7) the University's Associate Vice President of Student Affairs. The purpose of the interviews was to explore issues around accessibility and inclusion faced by different members of the University community. Additional data collected during the PAR process included PAR team meeting transcripts, photos taken by one of the participants with a disability, researcher field notes and other documents recommended by the participants (i.e., University newspaper, brochures, posters).

In order to maintain confidentiality, pseudonyms have been used for all interview participants. Although each member of the research team agreed to use their real names in reference to their participation on the research team, pseudonyms were given to them when using data gathered from their personal interviews. Sometimes participants referred to other individuals by first name. In these instances, a pseudonym was provided for that individual within the quote. In instances where participants were referring to members of the research team, such as Barry Wheeler or Pat Richards, a pseudonym was not used as per their suggestion. Another concern was that the identity of some of the participants, specifically staff members with specific job titles, may be deduced because of the use of their title. As such, staff members were asked how they would like to be referred to throughout the study. Two asked for their titles to be omitted from this paper, while three of the participants felt comfortable using their titles.

Data analysis was a continual process that began from the start of data collection (Arai and Pedlar 1997). Data were continually assessed, shared and reflected upon at team meetings. Transcript data were stored and coded using NVivo software. Initial codes were examined for common patterns which were then clustered together into broader categories. By organizing data into patterns and categories, we were able to uncover principal themes that related to our study's objectives (Arai and Pedlar 1997; Judah and Richardson 2006). Upon analysing the data, a five page outline of framework for creating a campus culture of inclusion emerged. This draft was shared with members of the research team and all of the research participants in order to solicit their reflections and comments. Participants were also invited to share insights at a focus group. Final suggestions and recommendations from the focus group and team meetings solidified the creation of a framework for creating a campus culture of inclusion.

A framework for creating a campus culture of inclusion

As the PAR team worked through the analysis of the data, they struggled with how best to organize the data into a resulting framework. We shared with them an existing framework focused on supporting the development of dementia-friendly communities called the Alzheimer's Disease and Related Dementias (ADRD) Planning Framework (Dupuis 2010), which drew on the social model of disability in its development. PAR members found the structure of the framework a helpful heuristic in critically reflecting on the important components of a campus culture of inclusion emerging from project data and, perhaps more importantly, as a useful structure for organizing their own data. Using the ADRD Planning Framework structure, the PAR team was able to reflect on what our emerging themes told us about what principles, pillars or foundational characteristics, and support mechanisms needed to be in place to create a campus culture of inclusion. What emerged from the data was our framework comprised of six guiding principles, three fundamental characteristics and six process pieces critical to the development of a campus culture that is inclusive of all community members, particularly persons with disabilities.

Guiding principles

In analysing the data, the PAR team came to realize that each setting within the campus community, and the people within it, are unique and therefore, a one-size fits all approach to inclusion would not work. As such, the team used the data to develop guiding principles, or core values, that would help community members guide their decision-making process and their actions towards creating an inclusive campus community, regardless of the specific community context. The framework includes six guiding principles: (1) access for all, (2) value the diversity and uniqueness of all, (3) value interdependence and social responsibility, (4) value diverse knowledge bases, voices and perspectives, (5) value the power of learning and education as tools for growth and change and (6) value the whole person.

Principle 1: access for all

The first principle, access for all, involves a commitment to identify and alleviate physical, social and systemic obstructions to meaningful community engagement. People access programmes, services or spaces in different ways; thus, accessibility works to ensure that everyone has equal opportunities to achieve well-being. Although not every person's needs may be met using universal standards of accessibility, what is important is that processes are in place to both systemically and individually accommodate needs. As Pat, the Coordinator for the Lifestyle and Fitness programs at the University stated '[Accessibility] doesn't just mean physical access, it means breaking down barriers… Access means you're thinking about the barriers that need to be removed to provide access'.

Principle 2: value the diversity and uniqueness of all

An inclusive campus community values the diversity and uniqueness in all and does not use personal characteristics as the basis for oppression or exclusion. Valuing diversity and uniqueness means that people are not just accommodated, but are seen as valuable members of the community where uniqueness and diversity are woven into the fabric of the community. People are seen as holistic beings with many facets to their identity. As

Carla, a student with a disability stated, 'A huge part of my identity is in realizing that my disability is only one facet of who I am and there's so many others that kind of take over from that'.

Principle 3: value interdependence and social responsibility

Communities that value interdependence and social responsibility genuinely want to help others, because they feel that they have a responsibility to those around them. This can be achieved by providing opportunities for community members to become aware of the plights of others and by fostering a culture of universal responsibility, leadership and volunteerism. This principle moves away from traditional notions of 'dependency' by encouraging the development of mutually supportive partnerships. As Beth, the Associate Vice President of Student Affairs, stated, 'I think that if you come from that core, it doesn't matter if you're a person of colour, a person with a disability, or white middle class kind of whatever, there's this sense that, we're part of a team so we need to look out for each other'.

Principle 4: value diverse knowledge bases, voices and perspectives

Strong partnerships within the community can only develop when the diverse knowledge bases, voices and perspectives are valued and incorporated in decision-making. It is essential for all community members, particularly those in positions of power, to actively respond to the ideas, perspectives and viewpoints of others. This is achieved when persons representing various stakeholder groups are meaningfully included on committees, organizations or advisory groups.

Principle 5: value the power of learning and education as tools for growth and change

All members of an inclusive campus community value the power of learning and education as a tool for growth and change. Formal and informal education opportunities help members broaden their awareness of relevant issues to create positive change. Learning extends beyond the classroom and is related to all aspects of campus life. Social and extra-curricular opportunities create avenues for community members to learn and share with one another. As James, a university alumnus with a disability, stated: 'University holds a lot of the best learning and it really happens outside of the classroom and it's going to make it better for everyone if that kind of culture is developed'.

Principle 6: value the whole person

In an inclusive campus community, the whole person is valued. Universities are not just spaces where people learn; they are places where they live, work, eat, play, socialize and develop. As Carla, a fourth year student with a disability, stated: 'school [university] is not just school. School is four years of life that preferably would be, you know, enjoyable and conducive to personality development as well as academic success'. Opportunities for physical activity, leisure, social interaction, meaningful engagements and personal development are a critical component of wellness and quality of life. The well-rounded person thrives, because they are connected to others, they develop new skills and they maintain a balance within life. Therefore, inclusive campus communities cater to the various functions that they serve and provide services and programmes that meet the complex needs of community members. A student who is living with depression, for

Table 1. Three characteristics of an inclusive campus community.

An Interconnected campus community	A supportive and enabling campus community	an informed campus community
• Fosters top-down and bottom-up connections • Develops synergistic campus partnerships	• Ensures the campus is physically accessible • Builds a community that is safe, supportive and welcoming • Provides opportunities to build social connections and personal development	• Continually learns about the needs and preferences of community members • Effectively informs the community of programmes and services • Provides learning opportunities for the community • Ensures service providers are informed, trained and qualified

example, would benefit from being connected to a web of support including the counselling office, the department of athletics and the centre for persons with disabilities in a manner that is seamless and easy to navigate, regardless of the point of entry.

Characteristics of a campus culture of inclusion

Several iterations of analysis of all of our data revealed three main characteristics that work together to create a campus culture of inclusion. These characteristics are the building blocks, or strong foundational pieces, required for constructing a campus that is supportive, accessible and welcoming to all citizens. These three characteristics are: (1) an Interconnected Campus Community, (2) a Supportive and Enabling Campus Community, and (3) an Informed Campus Community. This section will explore each of these characteristics. While each characteristic is presented as a distinct category, it is important to note that these characteristics are intertwined, interconnected and dependent on one another (Table 1).

An interconnected campus community

The lives of campus community members are often entwined and inter-reliant, thus requiring an interconnected campus community. This section explores the importance of: (1) fostering top-down and bottom-up interconnections, and (2) developing synergistic partnerships both within and outside of the university.

The first component of an interconnected campus community is the development of strong working relationships between those who hold the power to create, regulate and enforce policies, and those who are most affected by them. Major decision makers, who are committed to positive social change, actively listen to, and connect with, community members in a variety of ways to fully understand their needs and interests. These leaders work with the community to help shape an inclusive and welcoming environment while providing the accountability and enforcement necessary to enact change or follow through with recommendations. This collaborative approach builds working relationships between persons within all levels of the community. Gareth, a student and part-time staff member with the Department of Athletics, speaks to this process:

> Just having a culture like that established is important. You know, change in a workplace environment can be a really challenging endeavour but having all the supervisors definitely in line and having the same message and just treating people with respect and dignity and

caring about people…So having the supervisors really hammering that message into the staff I think is also really helpful…Just building a culture of accessibility and caring. Pat [supervisor] definitely thinks that caring about people is important and anybody she works with gets that impression. It just rubs off on you.

It is also important to acknowledge the role that middle managers and staff play to help connect decision makers to those who are impacted by decisions. These individuals strive to support students while following the policies mandated by their supervisors. Maintenance of strong connections and healthy working relationships between staff and major decision makers will enable staff to feel comfortable bringing issues forward on the students' behalf and will help them better understand the system within which they are working. Colleen, a staff member who recently acquired a disability, elaborated: 'We can't forget about that middle group because they're very influential because they are the ones that hear the cries for help and proposals for new initiatives and…they're getting often opposing pressures'.

Although staff and major decision makers play a substantial role in creating a campus culture of inclusion, the role that individuals and grass roots initiatives have on shaping a campus culture cannot be overstated. These individuals have an insider perspective on how the community can meet needs and preferences. It is essential for campus members to engage with campus-wide groups or committees in order to advocate for what they need and shape the university culture. As Beth stated:

It [initiatives around accessibility] doesn't come from [the president]. It's being driven by the Centre for Students with Disabilities. It's being pushed up…There has been a huge culture shift, right, and that's not all us. A lot of that is also coming from society…Students are coming up through schools now and being accommodated and learning to advocate better so some of it is coming naturally as well…And I think that's what builds it. It's gotta come from the top but it's gotta be supported at the bottom.

Another component of an interconnected campus community is the development of synergistic partnerships within and outside of the post-secondary community. A synergistic partnership approach occurs 'when individuals come together and collectively use their wealth of abilities and strengths to come up with a combined solution or response that often far exceeds what any one individual could come up with' (Dupuis et al. 2008, 21). Offices that support student success and well-being play an integral role in creating a culture of inclusion and therefore require strong working relationships between them. A collaborative approach to service provision creates an interconnected web of support that is proactive, holistic and seamless. It further enables staff to appropriately direct students to necessary resources and supports while taking their needs into account during program planning or policy development. Building connections within a large campus can be challenging, but can be fostered through inter-departmental training sessions, socials or resource fairs where various departments learn and share with each other about available resources and services. As Sidney, a staff member from the CSD, stated:

It all comes down to relationships. Do people know about the information? Do they know how to ask us things? Do they know who they can connect with about anything, any barriers that they might experience…It's a constant, you know, reconnecting with people, building those relationships with services and different people in those services, so then we can navigate it when we need to.

Campus communities are strengthened by the connections and partnerships they foster with those outside of their immediate community. The sharing of resources and infrastructures can save money, reduce inefficiencies and redundancies, enhance services and provide programmes that may otherwise not be available. Programmes that are open to both university and wider community members provide increased promotional opportunities which can generate extra income and garner community support. Post-secondary institutions that are connected to high schools will make for a more seamless transition into university, which can ultimately enable students to be more engaged in campus life. Moreover, students using satellite services or web-based learning options benefit from access to community resources or programmes. Sidney elaborated:

> The University is not an island unto itself. I think sometimes students, faculty, staff, start thinking about that because to a very large degree a lot of your needs can be met on campus, you know. But we are part of a larger community. There are a lot of other resources available in the community that aren't available on campus. And again that's a real challenge for each and every staff person, to kind of go above and beyond what's actually happening here to the broader community as well. But the reality is students live in the community.

A supportive and enabling campus community

An inclusive post-secondary community is supportive and enabling by considering the physical, psychological and social needs of its members. This enables all campus members to be engaged in campus life. This section examines how compassionate post-secondary communities can become supportive and enabling to all of its members by: (1) ensuring that the campus is physically accessible, (2) being a safe, supportive and welcoming environment and (3) providing a variety of opportunities to be engaged.

The experiences of participants revealed how inaccessible or unwelcoming environments directly resulted in their exclusion. One component of a supportive and enabling campus community is ensuring that the environment is physically accessible. Inclusive campus communities adhere to, and go above, mandated accessibility standards because they realize that accessibility is a key component of being inclusive. It is nearly impossible for social connections and personal development to occur when segments of the population are excluded from various aspects of community life. Participants noted how the physical space of an environment can be enhanced by implementing simple features such as push door buttons, ramps, accessible crosswalks and stable walking surfaces. In Canada, adequate and timely snow removal is particularly important and services that support students who need mobility assistance in the snow should be offered. The findings revealed that persons with disabilities are often subjected to environments that are unsafe or uncomfortable which limit their inclusion and engagement within the campus. Space is needed to manoeuvre around a room or building, environments need to be clutter-free and emergency exits need to be clearly marked. An accessible environment is more than getting into the front door. An accessible residence, for example, would ensure that students are able to freely access all public areas within the space, including the lounge or social areas. Natalie, an undergraduate student with cerebral palsy, spoke to the importance of accessibility:

> The basic accessibility issues need to be targeted first before you can make somebody feel included. Because for someone to feel like, included, they have to be able to get to the location or wherever they're going, right? And so like ramps or elevators or whatever you're gonna put it, that's what would need to be done first. And I think that's the thing I would tell schools [universities] wherever is not to underestimate people because if you build it they

would come, as corny as it sounds right? And as much as we may say "it's fine, it doesn't matter", it does matter.

Although physical accessibility is a key factor for inclusion, accessibility means different things to different people and is often not enough. As Colleen, a staff member with a physical disability, stated:

> When you talk about accessibility, do you mean getting in the front door? Do you mean getting beyond the front door and getting into a change room? Do you mean getting from the washroom and then into a programme? Do you mean getting into a programme that is indeed tailored to people with physical disabilities? And it's interesting; everybody has a different perception of accessibility. So in many people's mind, just getting through the front door is the critical piece. And it is, obviously, a critical piece. But I mean, not having the right programme is equally critical. What good is it to get through the front door if you then can't go to the washroom?…The facility is only the start. If you can't get through the front door, problem one, but the list of problems can be so long.

Our data emphasized the importance of addressing social barriers to inclusion. Just because one can enter the front door does not mean they will be treated fairly and equitably once they enter. A campus community of inclusion must also be supportive, welcoming, open-minded and comfortable for all people of diverse abilities. As Carla, a student with a disability, stated, 'You don't need physical accessibility when you have people that are open minded enough to make it accessible to you'. A safe and welcoming campus environment is created when people work towards a shared goal of inclusion. It occurs when members, particularly persons in positions of power, think and speak with sensitivity and act in ways that make others feel welcomed and included. Promoting issues that are important to persons of diverse backgrounds and abilities helps to increase the sensitivity towards, and understanding of, individuals within a community. The visibility of diversity within a community is also critical to creating a space that is welcoming and inclusive. Participants with disabilities noted how a visibly diverse environment helps to reduce the stigma and 'otherness' often associated with having a disability. As Natalie described:

> When I came [to this university] the first day, I walked into a lecture and I actually took my scooter to class and I remember thinking 'oh God, everyone's gonna be looking' and I looked up and no one cared. I sat down beside a girl and she started talking to me…Here I've never felt like riding a scooter was odd, I guess 'cause the students see it more often.…I've noticed other people riding scooters and which was not something you would of seen at [her previous university]. Everybody knew me because I was the girl that rides the scooter…Part of the reason that I left is 'cause I got tired of being 'that' girl.

Another participant noted how important it is for others to witness the realities and lives of persons with disabilities or differences, because it helps to increase awareness and create an inclusive culture where each individual is viewed as capable.

Another component of a supportive and enabling community is the provision of opportunities that build social connections and enhance personal development. Several students with disabilities commented on how they felt socially isolated when they began university and how this lack of connection was a reason why they did not want to participate in campus life. Many participants stated that they were more likely to be involved in campus life once they built social connections. Opportunities for recreation, leisure and other social engagements are essential because they foster personal development, well-being and social cohesion and support.

Participants told stories that demonstrated how socialization among diverse individuals (i.e., persons of different abilities, genders and nationalities) helped citizens to unlearn many harmful stigmas and assumptions and relearn a new appreciation for diversity and uniqueness. As such, community members require access to a variety of recreation and leisure opportunities that meets their needs and preferences. While this will include recreation programmes and wellness initiatives, many participants spoke of the informal activities that they took part in such as going to coffee shops, pubs and bars on campus. Participants encouraged campus communities to think outside of the traditional sports and recreation programming and try new ways of engaging persons. These informal activities and events are a great way for people to get involved, meet others and build social connections.

Programme planners can support participation by offering a blend of social, solitary, active and spectator options, ensuring that all campus spaces (including spectator areas, concession stands and washrooms) are accessible and that students are provided with the supports and resources necessary to participate. Students with mental health issues, for example, identified to their student advisor at the CSD that they felt overwhelmed by the noise and crowds during orientation week, which posed a barrier to participation. In response, the university offers a variety of orientation activities that include low crowd and quiet options. Another strength of this campus was that students were supported by the CSD in matters beyond the academic. CSD advisors would support students in achieving their social, personal and recreational needs. As Sidney, a staff member of the CSD, explained:

> There might be time at the end of the appointment to talk about other stuff... You know, 'how do you balance your life'? 'What other things are involved in your life'? ... 'what do you do'? 'What places do you access here on campus in order to connect with recreational groups or activities'?

Service providers can work collaboratively with the students to develop programmes that meet the specific needs of those not met in general programming. Specialized or targeted programs can enable participants to be with others who share a similar situation or ability level. However, they can further seclude persons who are already marginalized, and people may not feel comfortable being grouped with others who simply share a similar ability level.

An informed campus community

The data revealed how critical it is for all members within a campus community to become informed. Not only do service providers and programme planners need to become informed on the needs and interests of community members, but community members themselves need access to information that can enhance their health and well-being. Our data points to four key areas related to an informed campus community: (1) continually learns about the needs and preferences of community members, (2) effectively informs the community of programmes and services, (3) provides learning opportunities for the community, and (4) ensures service providers are informed, trained and qualified.

The first component of an Informed Community relates to the need for decision makers to continually seek out and gather information concerning the needs and preferences of community members in order to provide responsive services and programs. Various channels to solicit input or feedback on programmes and services are critical. These feedback channels can be systematic and formal, such as the use of advisory committees or councils, or informal, including the development and mainten-ance of strong working relationships between community members and service providers. It is important for community members to be informed on these feedback mechanisms and for them to be accessible. The process of asking community members, directly, what they want and need opens up lines of communication and ensures that programmes or services are based on the community's genuine needs and interests. As Natalie, an undergraduate student with a physical disability, stated:

> See what they like, what they don't like and make suggestions, because nothing can hurt from asking…If somebody asked me my true opinion I would respect them so much more for it because if they guess that I decide not to go to the pool because of this, this and this, most of the time they're wrong because they're not in my head. So it's better just to ask it and not beat around it because if you beat around it, it makes it worse.

Second, data revealed that community members require information on programmes and services through the use of effective promotional strategies that are intuitive, easy-to-navigate and accessible. This is important since persons with disabilities are often denied access to information either because information is provided in a format that does not meet their needs and preferences or because of systemic oppression. Therefore, post-secondary institutions need to consider, and cater to, the variety of ways that people access and receive information. Promotional materials in a variety of formats, including online, in print, word-of-mouth, Braille or large font, make it easy for students, staff and others to be involved. Marketing strategies that target specific populations are sometimes necessary to inform them that facilities and/or programmes can meet their needs. The physical location of where information is provided should take into account the varied needs and preferences of students. For example, participants noted how information booths in the student centre may be an effective strategy to inform students of recreation opportunities. However, such a crowded space may not be accessible to persons with mobility impairments or mental health issues. Indicating the accessibility of an event (including information on different accessibility options) on promotional materials enables people to know ahead of time if the event will be appropriate for them. Service providers can also make it known that accommodation is available upon request. Of course, the most effective way of uncovering how best to share information about programmes and services is by asking students with disabilities: what are the best methods for getting information into their hands.

Another aspect of an informed community is the provision of learning opportunities for the community to learn and share with each other in a variety of ways. For example, students with disabilities often mentioned how they do not feel entitled to recreation or leisure, particularly when they are struggling to keep up with school work. As Carla, a student with a physical disability, stated:

> I don't know who would do this but somebody coming in and letting people with disabilities know that it's okay that you don't have to spend 24 hours a day on schoolwork just because it takes you longer. Like, you're entitled to the breaks that other people are entitled to too…I feel as though a lot of students with disabilities are willing to forego these things.

Participants noted the value of receiving information from trusted sources (such as advisors, parents and teachers) about the importance of addressing their various needs (social, emotional, physical and intellectual) in order to achieve a well-balanced life. It was suggested that healthy living options could be promoted through a variety of ways, including educational series, networking sessions, mentorships or support groups.

Universities can also provide opportunities for campus members to become informed about the lives of those who make up the community through awareness campaigns, story sharing, simulated activities or various media outlets. As identified by participants, experiential learning and sharing between diverse groups of people played a major role in breaking down the stigma and prejudices that often exist around diversity. As James, a former varsity track athlete with a visual impairment, indicated: much of the exclusion that he encountered on the track team was a result of others not being informed about the realities of his disability:

> I think it [exclusion on the track team] mainly came down to just people not being sure and not really knowing as opposed to not, like not wanting to help me, adamantly against helping me. Just a lack of information or education doesn't really help. And partly from my point of view because as a first year student, you know, it took a while for me to really learn to ask for what I needed and to ask for help, I think, and that was sort of part of it too.

The last component of an informed community is to ensure that service providers are informed, trained and qualified. Issues of diversity and inclusiveness are the responsibility of the entire community. A campus culture of inclusion is possible when all staff members, faculty, coaches and service providers are trained on diversity awareness and sensitivity, as well as the policies and procedures that are in place to support persons with disabilities or alternative needs. Students will benefit from having faculty members who are informed on how to work with them and on-campus supports to overcome learning obstacles and facilitate a welcoming environment. Service providers and programmers can develop systems that facilitate inclusion and accessibility in the form of policies, procedures or protocols which are shared with all involved persons. This ensures consistency of services and that processes are in place to meet needs. It also ensures that there is consistent and reliable information being given to those who inquire and that people are able to access services and programmes with ease and relative independence. Qualified staff members who are specifically trained and certified to cater to the special needs of community members, such as in the fitness centre, are critical. An inclusive environment that supports people as just a part of 'business as usual' reduces the stigmas associated with accommodations, and it facilitates a consistently welcoming environment. Pamela, a senior staff member in the Department of Athletics, indicated that training sessions can help staff members become more aware of, and open to, issues of diversity and inclusion which will help them be more sensitive to those who may need assistance:

> All of our fitness personnel are trained around openness and inclusiveness...They also have training around eating disorders and what to do if this happens. So if somebody blind shows up to their [fitness] class, they get training enough philosophically to say you're there for them too and then they know that they need to come down and talk to me. And if that's the case, we get them a volunteer.

Putting the framework into action

Creating a campus culture of inclusion may not be an easy endeavour, as several participants cautioned that social change within a university is complex and can take much time and resources. They also noted how culture change within a university context requires patience, problem-solving skills, commitment and a willingness to move towards a shared vision for the future. However, a student with a disability said it best: 'Obstacles are only obstacles when there are no other options. And there's always other options, some are just not developed yet' (Carla).

This section provides the 'how to' piece by offering practical strategies on how a culture of inclusion can be collectively developed. Participants identified the following six process pieces for fuelling and sustaining a campus culture of inclusion over time: (1) create a vision for the future, (2) construct a plan to achieve the vision, (3) secure funds to put the plan in place, (4) be proactive to make change happen, (5) reach beyond compliance and (6) think critically and measure actions against the vision.

First, post-secondary institutions seeking to create a campus culture of inclusion can collaborate with campus community members to create a shared vision for the future which will shape how the community develops. This vision, along with the campus' guiding principles, will strengthen the culture by guiding decisions and actions, clarifying priorities and attracting individuals who align themselves with similar values.

Once a vision is created, then one must construct a clear plan to achieve the vision. This can involve systematically and deliberately weaving the vision into the fabric of the campus community, including curricula, extra-curricular, programme planning and the development of support services. This approach yields the additional benefit of developing students who come to reflect the university's values by witnessing them in action and by being engaged in social issues that relate to them.

The third process involves securing funding to carry out the plan. Systematically working physical and social accessibility improvements into yearly budgets will provide a consistent funding base and ensure accessibility features are considered upfront. It may be helpful to move towards a system where resources are allocated based on the university's overall strategic plan and vision. This involves considering how life can be enhanced for those within and beyond the university and then determining where resources need to be allocated to accomplish that vision.

The fourth process piece for creating an inclusive campus community is remaining proactive to make change happen. Accessibility and inclusion will become part of the everyday culture when programmes, services and spaces proactively consider the diverse needs and abilities of the campus community. This involves being aware of current issues or challenges facing community members and anticipating and removing barriers before accommodations are requested. Being proactive in creating an inclusive community can also yield cost savings since retro-fitting adjustments for accessibility is usually much more expensive and people-intensive (Wentz, Jaeger, and Lazar 2011).While there may need to be an initial investment in accessibility, costs will be reduced over time.

The fifth process piece is reaching beyond compliance. It is essential for post-secondary institutions to act in accordance with current legislations and to recognize that a community is enhanced when people are treated fairly and equitably. Considerations should be made to ensure that all community members have the opportunity to meaningfully participate in all aspects of community life and not just because it is mandated by law but because they truly believe that all people matter. An environment is more welcoming, warm and strengthened when a community goes beyond compliance and moves towards building a culture of genuine compassion and inclusion.

Last, in order to maintain an inclusive campus community, it is important for the community to think critically and measure actions against the vision. This enables communities to solve problems creatively, evaluate current programs or services and plan for the future. It is useful to routinely question the way things are, how they got to be that way, who benefits from the way things are, who is excluded or oppressed and how things can be improved.

Conclusion

The study's findings are derived from the personal experiences of those within one university community; thus, additional research could broaden our understanding of this topic, particularly from various demographic or geographic contexts. Other universities, globally, may want to use the same process to understand how they can include all citizens in higher education and, in doing so, engage in a participatory process that serves to empower all key stakeholders. Nonetheless, this framework has enormous implications for practice in terms of informing what is necessary for creating and sustaining inclusive communities. Although this framework specifically explores how post-secondary institutions can support engagement in all areas of campus life, components of this framework can be used to encourage universities, and other communities, to collaborate and create community conversations that raise awareness of each other's perspectives and work towards collective problem solving, particularly around issues of inclusion and accessibility. It encourages individuals to consider how their actions, both passive and active, either cause suffering or enable people to thrive, while replacing indifference with care and concern (Williams 2008). The framework can serve as a starting point for dialogue around these issues while providing the factors necessary for putting this framework into action. The research also sheds light on the process by which university stakeholders, or community members, can use PAR approaches to unite relevant individuals in order to achieve a common goal.

It is understood that by facilitating educational opportunities for people with disabilities we are creating citizens who are better able to contribute towards, and participate in, all aspects of civic life, including employment. This ultimately helps to create communities where citizens are better able to be productive contributors to communities and economies. However, the findings from this study demonstrate that post-secondary institutions are also creating inclusive campus communities, because they are guided by a genuine desire to value and support all community members. This approach to inclusion creates a culture where community members are interdependent and accountable to one another. This supports the underpinnings of critical disability theory where disability is seen as an inherent part of society, and thus, the responsibility to ameliorate the challenges faced by disability is shared. It also supports critical disability theorists who would argue that 'how disability is perceived, diagnosed, and treated, scientifically and socially, is reflected in assumptions about the social responsibility towards people with disabilities as a group' (Rioux 2003, 289).

Communities, organizations and even governments are recognizing the need for accessible and welcoming communities, as indicated by the rapid emergence of age-friendly, healthy and livable communities (Public Health Agency of Canada 2011; World Health Organization 2011). Such initiatives are creating a movement that is shifting how we perceive each other, and ultimately how we care for one another. This movement encourages communities to strive toward 'the development and sustenance of social conditions within which all persons have the greatest opportunity to realise their potentialities, both as unique individuals and as members of great communities and societies' (Williams 2008, 7–8). This involves creating a culture where community members are sensitive to the needs and interests of each other, because there is an understanding that one's successes and failures are connected with that of others

(Williams 2008). According to Williams (2008), social justice and human flourishing can only occur when citizens develop meaningful relationships with one another and become aware of the interdependence that exists among us. Without this basis, injustices such as exclusion, harm and suffering will continue. As Kaufman (2003) stated, 'By working to transform the structures of the institutions we are part of, we make those institutions serve the needs of everyone, and we stop oppressive dynamics from being reproduced' (297). Combating this oppression will require systemic changes and a reconceptualization of what is important to community, and to society as a whole. Larger social change will require serious reflection about what we value as a society and how we can better consider the needs of all citizens. If communities use this framework to create cultures of inclusion, what will this mean to citizens? What might our communities look like? Clair, a student with a disability, explained what this would look like to her:

> An accessible world - anywhere that would help me not to notice my disability, not in a sense that I'm not comfortable with it but in the sense that I want to be so comfortable that it doesn't cause me any differences…I like when my disability doesn't necessarily enter the equation…So like if there's a ramp right beside the staircase then the staircase isn't going to bother me…For me, the perfect world would be one in which my disability causes no obstacles. The more obstacles we can eliminate the happier I'll be.

Notes on contributors

Jennifer Gillies, PhD., Executive Director, Alzheimer Societies of Kitchener-Waterloo and Cambridge 831 Frederick Street Kitchener, Ontario N2B 2B4. Email: jlgillies@alzheimerkw.com

Sherry L. Dupuis, PhD., Professor, Department of Recreation and Leisure Studies, 200 University Avenue, Waterloo, Ontario N2V 3G1. Email: ldupuis@uwaterloo.ca

References

Arai, S., and A. Pedlar. 1997. "Building Communities through Leisure: Citizen Participation in a Healthy Community." *Journal of Leisure Research* 29 (2): 167–182.

Ashton-Shaeffer, C., H. Gibson, C. Autry, and C. Hanson. 2001. "Meaning of Sport to Adults with Physical Disabilities: A Disability Sport Camp Experience." *Sociology of Sport Journal* 18: 95–114.

Blinde, E., and L. McClung. 1997. "Enhancing the Physical and Social Self Through Recreational Activity: Accounts of Individuals with Physical Disabilities." *Adapted Physical Activity Quarterly* 14: 327–344.

Blinde, E., and D. Taub. 1999. "Personal Empowerment through Sport and Physical Activity: Perspectives from Male College Students with Physical and Sensory Disabilities." *Journal of Sport Behavior* 22 (2): 181–199.

Dattel, L. (2012, September 10). "90 Million Budgeted to Improve Disabled Access at Universities and Colleges." *Harretz*, p. 1. Accessed July 7, 2013. http://www.haaretz.com/business/nis-90-million-budgeted-to-improve-disabled-access-at-universities-and-colleges.premium-1.468789.

Department of Justice Canada. 1982. *Canadian Charter of Rights and Freedoms*. Accessed July 7, 2013. http://laws.justice.gc.ca/en/charter/.

DePauw, K. P. 1997. "The (In)visibility of Disability: Cultural Contexts and 'Sporting Bodies'." *Quest* 49 (4): 416–430. doi:10.1080/00336297.1997.10484258

DePauw, K., and S. Gavron. 2005. *Disability and Sport*. Champaign, IL: Human Kinetics.

Devlin, R., and D. Pothier. 2006. "Introduction: Toward a Critical Theory of Dis-citizenship." In *Critical Disability Theory: Essays in Philosophy, Politics, Policy and Law*, edited by R. Devlin and D. Pothier, 1–22. Vancouver, BC: BC Press.

Dupuis, S., J. Gillies, A. Mantle, L. Loiselle, and L. Sadler. 2008. *Creating Partnerships in Dementia Care: A Changing Melody Toolkit*. Waterloo, ON: MAREP, University of Waterloo.

Dupuis, S. 2010. "Improving the Lives of Persons With Dementia and Their Families through Enhancing Social Policy, Leisure Policy, and Practice." In *Decentring Work*, edited by H. Mail, S. Aria, and D. Reid, 91–117. Alberta: University of Calgary press.

Duquette, C. 2000. "Experiences at University: Perceptions of Students with Disabilities." *The Canadian Journal of Higher Education* 30 (2): 123–142.

Gillies, J. 2005. "Campus Athletic Opportunities for University Students with Disabilities: Is it their Right?" Major Research Paper. Toronto, Ontario: York University.

Gillies, J. 2012. "Critical Disability Theory." In *Encyclopedia of Quality of Life Research*, edited by A. Michalos, 1st ed. Springer.

Hughes, B., and K. Paterson. 1997. "The Social Model of Disability and the Disappearing Body: Towards a Sociology of Impairment." *Disability & Society* 12 (3): 325–340. doi:10.1080/09687599727209.

Judah, M.-L., and G. Richardson. 2006. "Between a Rock and a (Very) Hard Place: The Ambiguous Promise of Action Research in the Context of State Mandated Teacher Professional Development." *Action Research* 4 (1): 65–80. doi:10.1177/1476750306060543.

Kaufman, C. 2003. *Ideas for Action: Relevant Theory for Radical Change*. Cambridge, MA: South End Press.

Legislative Assembly of Ontario. 2004. *Bill 118, An Act Respecting the Development, Implementation and Enforcement of Standards Relating to Accessibility with Respect to Goods, Services, Facilities, Employment, Accommodation, Buildings and all other things Specified in the Act for Persons with Disabilities*. Accessed July 7, 2013. http://www.ontla.on.ca/web/committee-proceedings/committee_transcripts_details.do?DocumentID=22320&Date=2005-02-28&ParlCommID=7430&BillID=308&Business=&locale=en&detailPage=%2Fcommittee-pro-ceedings%2Ftranscripts%2Ffiles_html%2F28-FEB-2005_SP022.htm.

Merchant, D., and A. Gajar. 1997. "A Review of the Literature on Self-Advocacy Components in Transition Programmes for Students with Learning Disabilities." *Journal of Vocational Rehabilitation* 8: 223–231. doi:10.1016/S1052-2263(97)00005-6.

Oliver, M. 1993. "Re-defining Disability: A Challenge to Research." In *Disabling Barriers — Enabling Environments*, edited by J. Swain, V. Finkelstein, S. French, and M. Oliver, 61–68. Buckingham: Open University Press.

Ontario Ministry of Community and Social Services. 2008. *Access On: Making Ontario Accessible*. Accessed July 7, 2013. http://www.mcss.gov.on.ca/en/mcss/programs/accessibility/index.aspx.

Promis, D., N. Erevelles, and J. Matthews. 2001. "Re-conceptualizing Inclusion: The Politics of University Sports and Recreation Programmes for Students with Mobility Impairments." *Sociology of Sport Journal* 18: 37–50.

Public Health Agency of Canada. 2011. *Age Friendly Communities Initiative*. Accessed July 7, 2013. http://www.phac-aspc.gc.ca/sh-sa/ifa-fiv/2008/initiative-eng.php.

Rioux, M. 2003. "On Second Thought: Constructing Knowledge, Law, Disability, and Inequality." In *The Human Rights of Persons with Intellectual Disabilities: Different but Equal*, edited by S. Herr, L. Gostin, and H. Koh, 287–317. Don Mills, ON: Oxford University Press.

Rioux, H. M., and C. Frazee. 1999. "The Canadian Framework for Disability Equality Rights." In *Disability, Divers-ability, and Legal Change*, edited by M. Jones and L. A. Basser Marks, 171–187. Boston, MA: M. Nijhoff Publishers.

Rioux, H. M., and M. Prince. 2002. "The Canadian Political Landscape of Disability: Policy Perspectives, Social Status, Interest Groups and the Rights Movement." In *Federalism, Democracy And Disability Policy In Canada*, edited by A. Putee, 11–29. Kingston: McGill-Queen's University.

South African Government Information. 2013. "Deputy Minister Advocates for Disability Compliance in South African Universities". Press Release. Accessed July 4, 2013. http://www.info.gov.za/speech/DynamicAction?pageid=461&sid=35608&tid=104069.

Taub, D., E. Blinde, and R. Greer. 1999. "Stigma Management through Participation in Sport and Physical Activity: Experiences of Male College Students with Physical Disabilities." *Human Relations* 52 (11): 1469–1483.

Turner, B. S. 2001. "Disability and the Sociology of The Body." In *Handbook of Disability Studies*, edited by G. L. Albrecht, K. D. Seelman, and M. Bury, 252–266. Thousand Oaks, CA: Sage Publications, Inc.

United Nations. 2006. *Convention on the Rights of Persons with Disabilities: About the Convention*. Accessed July 18, 2013. http://www.un.org/disabilities/convention/questions.shtml#ten

Wentz, B., P. Jaeger, and J. Lazar. 2011. "Retrofitting Accessibility: The Legal Inequality of After-the-Fact Online Access for Persons with Disabilities in the United States." *First Monday* 16 (11). Accessed July 7, 2013. http://firstmonday.org/ojs/index.php/fm/article/view/3666/3077.

Williams, C. R. 2008. "Compassion, Suffering and the Self: A Moral Psychology of Social Justice." *Current Sociology* 56 (1): 5–24. doi:10.1177/0011392107084376.

World Health Organization. 2011. *Global Age Friendly Communities: A Guide*. Accessed November 29, 2011. http://www.phac-aspc.gc.ca/sh-sa/ifa-fiv/2008/initiative-eng.php.

Zola, I. K. 1993. "Self, Identity and The Naming Question: Reflections on the Language of Disability." *Social Science and Medicine* 36 (2): 167–173. doi:10.1016/0277-9536(93)90208-L.

Using Photovoice to listen to adults with intellectual disabilities on being part of the community

Stuart J. Schleien[a], Lindsey Brake[a], Kimberly D. Miller[a] and Ginger Walton[b]

[a]Department of Community and Therapeutic Recreation, University of North Carolina at Greensboro, NC, USA; [b]The Arc of Greensboro, Greensboro, NC, US

Imagine if you were offered a glance through the lens of a very unique photographer: a member of your community who has an intellectual or developmental disability (ID/DD). A community-based participatory research method, Photovoice, was used to enable seven individuals with ID/DD the opportunity to document their lives through the use of photography and discuss their interests, hopes and dreams. Specifically, this methodology provided them with opportunities to share their concerns about their community access and communicate with the larger community using photographs and the collective ideas of the group. Common themes were revealed among the participants, including their hidden talents, community membership and sense of belonging, consumerism and making choices, desired independence, limited connections to the community and a desire to be treated as adults. Two themes – community membership and desire for independence – are expounded upon, as they appeared to be the most relevant to improving one's quality of life and greater self-determination.

Introduction

There have been numerous efforts in the past several decades to increase the participation and inclusion of people with intellectual and other developmental disabilities (ID/DD) in schools and community environments. These efforts and accomplishments have included self-advocacy and family member advocacy activities, legislative initiatives, development of new programmatic practices and innovative research pursuits. Additional support for increased community access has come from TASH (formerly The Association of Persons with Severe Handicaps) whose national agenda called for an expansion of inclusive educational, employment and community opportunities across the USA (Carter et al. 2012). Relatedly, the National Recreation and Park Association, through its Position Statement on Inclusion, made a clear statement on the value of inclusive service delivery to participants with and without disabilities in the USA (Schleien, Miller, and Shea 2009). Yet with all of these efforts to increase meaningful access to ongoing community activities, current research suggests that people with significant disabilities remain isolated from their peers without disabilities with community opportunities remaining unavailable (Anderson and Kress 2003; Carter et al. 2012; National Disability Rights Network 2011).

Consequently, individuals with ID/DD have restricted social networks that often consist of relationships with other people with a similar label, family members and staff members that are paid to work with them (Clement and Bigby 2009). As a result of this segregation, they have been excluded from full participation within their communities and remain one of the most physically and socially inactive and segregated groups in our communities (Zijlstra and Vlaskamp 2005).

Participating in recreation, sports and social activities with peers is an essential aspect of one's quality of life. Active, vital and socially connected people participate in a wide range of activities and places throughout their lifetime. Community recreation activities promote the learning of new skills; physical, mental and emotional health; provide opportunities for developing new relationships and making friends; and help individuals find a desirable balance between work and leisure (Sable and Gravink 2005; Schleien, Ray, and Green 1997). Although the benefits of inclusive recreation are clearly understood, and a variety of these services have been designed, there remains an abundance of community agencies that still do not practise inclusive services (Anderson and Kress 2003; Devine and King 2006; Miller, Schleien, and Lausier 2009; Schleien, Miller, and Shea 2009). In these cases, either programmes are not accessible to individuals with disabilities or segregated activities serving only people with similar disabilities are available.

To compound this problem, not only are individuals with ID/DD typically inactive and segregated, but they also have few opportunities to participate in decisions that affect their lives (Jurkowski 2008). In research studies, they are often employed as subjects rather than engaged as research participants (Horwitz et al. 2000; Paiewonsky 2011). Individuals with ID/DD are now seen as having unique and important views towards service delivery and available activities and are in need of a strong voice. Service providers cannot remain overly reliant on so-called 'experts' to make all the decisions concerning their livelihoods. What strategies and opportunities can be identified to empower these 'silenced' individuals to help create the change within the community for which society at large strives? Through Photovoice participatory action research, some of these answers may be provided by offering a glimpse into the ideas and perspectives of these self-advocates through the photography lens.

Literature review

Photovoice: what is it?

Photovoice is a creative form of community-based participatory research. Its roots are grounded in both qualitative and action research. Theoretical underpinnings for Photovoice include Frieri's (1973) critical education approach, feminist theory and documentary photography (Wang and Burris 1997). Friere's approach is to identify important issues in people's lives, to critically reflect on them through dialogue and to identify root causes and discuss potential solutions, and these form the foundations of the Photovoice methodology, with the exception of one critical detail. Friere provided visual images to those participating in the project, whereas in Photovoice, participants create their own images which could further empower participants. Feminist theory informs Photovoice methodology in its recognition that research may be biased by the dominant culture, and thus the need for individuals from underrepresented groups to serve as authorities of their own lives through methods that assert the value of their experiences. Finally, Photovoice draws on the critical consciousness that is raised through the powerful visual images generated through the practice of documentary photography.

Some of the initial Photovoice researchers defined it as a method of seeing the world from the viewpoint of people who are leading different lives (Wang and Burris 1994). Cameras are provided to members of underrepresented groups, and a 'voice' is created through the photographs that are taken. The viewpoints of these under-represented groups can be eye-opening since they often vary substantially from the typical and stereotyped viewpoints found in society.

Utilization of Photovoice

In the past, Photovoice has been used with a variety of populations with voices that have often gone unheard. People who are homeless (Wang, Cash, and Power 2000) and aboriginal breast cancer survivors (Poudrier and Mac-Lean 2009) are under-represented groups that have benefited from this 'technique that places the selected individuals in charge of documenting their lives' (Booth and Booth 2003, 432). Participants are also empowered to become community change agents while enhancing personal growth and social connections (Killion and Wang 2000). The Photovoice process usually contains three primary and complementary goals to benefit a number of segregated groups. These goals include enabling people to record and reflect upon their community's strengths and concerns; promoting critical dialogue and knowledge about important community issues through large and small group discussions of photographs; and reaching policy-makers and initiating change in the community (Wang and Burris 1997).

Individuals with ID/DD have become empowered by Photovoice, such as when Booth and Booth (2003) worked with mothers with learning disabilities to, 'challenge discriminatory views about this group of vulnerable families by narrowing the gap between how others see them and how they see themselves' (440). The researchers found that Photovoice was an effective means of revealing different perspectives for these underrepresented groups. To these researchers, Photovoice offered a method for 'grasping what is going on at the point in people's lives where biography and society intersect' (440).

The Photovoice methodology was implemented by Jurkowski and Paul-Ward (2007), Jurkowski (2008), and Jurkowski, Rivera and Hammel (2009) who worked with Latinos with ID on changing their perspectives on healthy living. They discovered that Photovoice 'enabled individuals with intellectual disabilities to express their real-life experiences through photographic images that represent their perspective as they interact in their environment' (Jurkowski 2008, 9). Through this initiative, Jurkowski, Rivera and Hammel (2009) found that Photovoice acted as an empowering tool that enabled photographers to reveal themes related to social relationships, emotional states, energy, interconnection between work and health, beliefs about healthy behaviour and culturally centred beliefs about health. Their findings were presented in a town hall meeting attended by service providers, community leaders, caregivers and people with disabilities. Meeting attendees discussed the findings and generated recommendations and action steps which were presented to agency administrators for use in future programme development (Jurkowski and Paul-Ward 2007).

Through her work with college students with ID, Paiewonsky (2011) adapted a combined methodology of Photovoice and a web-based digital storytelling technology called VoiceThread. Through this technology, college students developed, implemented and accomplished action steps as an integral part of their Photovoice project. The students' findings were presented to university partners and at conferences. They developed training materials for students, parents and professionals, as well as an online consortium of college options for individuals with ID.

Researchers have been encouraged by the success of this relatively new research methodology that is revealing new and different perspectives of individuals who had previously been marginalized from society. It is with this foundation in mind that we instigated this Photovoice study with two primary intentions: (a) to provide individuals with ID/DD a voice concerning their access, participation and inclusion in the community and (b) to attempt to instigate change in the community by sharing these voices with myriad audiences.

Methods

The Arc is a national grassroots organization comprising more than 700 state and local chapters across the USA, which started more than 60 years ago. The Arc's mission, in part, is to actively support community participation and inclusion of individuals with ID/DD. A local chapter of The Arc, located in a mid-size, southeastern city in the USA, reached out to a university research team with a desire to gain a better understanding from the perspective of their members with ID/DD of the barriers experienced and supports needed for increased community participation and inclusion. Through focus groups conducted by this collaborative team prior to the current study, a range of different perspectives were gained from self-advocates concerning their needs, wants and dreams to become more accepted and engaged within their communities. This research team believed Photovoice methodology aligned well with the desire to expound on these focus group results in a manner consistent with The Arc's promotion of self-advocacy among its constituents. A Photovoice initiative was implemented in 2011 to address the following research questions: (a) how do individuals with ID/DD perceive community access, participation and social inclusion? And (b) how does Photovoice inform community members about the inclusive community participation of individuals with ID/DD?

Phase one

The Photovoice project progressed through three discrete phases (see Figure 1). The initial phase began with preliminary and organizational tasks, as well as instructor training. Each participant was assigned to a single instructor that (s)he worked with throughout the entire project. Participants were selected based on their responses to an invitation letter from The Arc. This letter explained a number of important details including a description of the need for a committed 'assistant' who would be comfortable and willing to work with the participant throughout the Photovoice programme. Assistants were necessary due to their vital role of providing support in the technical aspects of utilizing digital cameras (e.g., need to recharge batteries and what to do if the wrong button was pushed), prompts to complete photography assignments, and transportation to and from programme meetings or photography

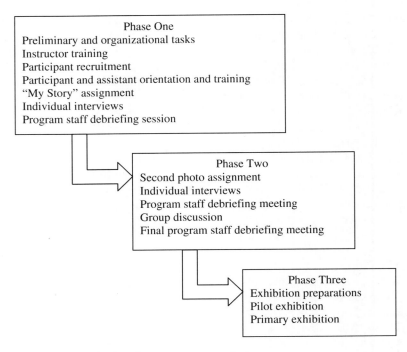

Phase One
Preliminary and organizational tasks
Instructor training
Participant recruitment
Participant and assistant orientation and training
"My Story" assignment
Individual interviews
Program staff debriefing session

Phase Two
Second photo assignment
Individual interviews
Program staff debriefing meeting
Group discussion
Final program staff debriefing meeting

Phase Three
Exhibition preparations
Pilot exhibition
Primary exhibition

Figure 1. Programme tasks for phases one, two and three.

locations. By clearly differentiating roles between the photographers and assistants, participants were empowered to share their personal perspectives, but with support available when necessary in order to do so.

A list of required meetings and events, along with a participant consent form, were other essential components of the invitation letter. Four criteria were established for the recruitment of participants for Photovoice. Participants had to be (a) 18 years of age or older, (b) a member of the local Arc, (c) able to demonstrate sufficient verbal communication skills to express meanings associated with their photographs and had to (d) demonstrate the ability to understand the consent process. A total of seven participants, all with mild to moderate ID, were engaged in the Photovoice initiative. Table 1 provides a brief description of the seven participants.

The second component of this first phase included holding a group meeting which all participants and assistants attended. The orientation began with a discussion of

Table 1. Photovoice participant demographics/characteristics.

Participant (pseudonym)	Age	Disability	Employment	Living arrangement	Photovoice assistant
Garrett	48	Intellectual disability	16 h/wk	With mother	Brother
Patrick	34	Down syndrome	8 h/wk	With parents	Father
Lisa	35	Intellectual disability	None	With mother	Mother
William	21	Intellectual disability	Student	College housing	Parents
Taylor	38	Intellectual disability	8 h/wk	With parents	Mother
Sam	32	Down syndrome	6 h/wk	With parents	Mother
David	26	Intellectual disability	8 h/wk	With parents	Father

Table 2. Differentiated roles of participants and assistants.

Participant	Assistant
Being responsible for camera	Providing assignment reminders to participant
Generating ideas for photos	Providing assistance only when necessary
Getting written consent from photo subjects	Appropriate assistance: support with camera operation; transportation; taking a photo when asked
Asking someone to take a photo if participant wanted to be in the photo	Inappropriate assistance: influencing what photos should be taken; speaking on behalf of participant during interviews

the programme goals and methods. A detailed explanation was provided to explain the differentiated roles of participants and their assistants and is depicted in Table 2.

The use of the digital camera was demonstrated with specific adaptations. A slide show was used to illustrate use of the digital camera and participants were walked through step-by-step instructions with their cameras in hand. Supplemental learning tools included a detailed list of camera instructions, a brief pocket-size set of camera instructions and a photo packet that displayed each button on the camera. These supplemental learning tools were provided to both the participants and assistants. Additional time was provided for the participants and their assistants to practise using their cameras after instruction was completed.

The ethics of photography and the importance of consent were discussed with the group, including the need to explain to potential photograph subjects why participants wished to take their picture, were asking for their permission, and were obtaining a signature of consent. The fact that some people may not want their photograph taken was also discussed. In order to minimize the reliance on communicative abilities, a pocket-sized photo-release booklet was provided to the participants, which provided a brief written explanation of the project, how the photos would be utilized and space to obtain signatures from individuals who the photographers desired to photograph. Towards the end of the meeting, the first assignment was introduced with a supplemental worksheet to assist the participants to organize their ideas. This 'My Story' assignment asked participants to take photos of people, places, and activities that were important to them. The participants were given two weeks to complete this assignment, with a 30-photo maximum.

The third component of phase one included a discussion between the instructor, participant and his/her assistant. Instructors reviewed the photos with each participant and allowed them to explain each of them in turn. During this process, the instructor noted several primary ideas the participant appeared to be communicating through their photographs. The instructor discussed these ideas with the participant and they were validated or altered based on the participant's feedback. The participant was then asked to choose the three ideas he/she felt were most important and one photo that best represented each idea. A series of prompts were used to discuss each of the three photos in further detail that included: Why did you take this photo?, What are the people, places and activities in this photo?, What do you like about these people, places and activities?, and What bothers you about these people, places and activities?

At times during these individual interviews, input was provided by the assistants. The interviewers managed this input by redirecting the conversation to the photographer and asking him/her to validate any ideas that may have been influenced by the assistant. Once the individual interviews were completed, programme staff (i.e. researchers, Community Resource Specialist of The Arc and instructors) held a debriefing meeting to discuss similarities, differences and themes across the participants' photos.

Phase two

Phase two resembled several of the steps within phase one, with a few exceptions. The instructors provided their respective participants and assistants with the next assignment through the participant's preferred method (i.e., face-to-face, phone call, text message or e-mail). Participants were asked to take new photos in response to the following two questions: what people, places and activities make you feel important and what are your skills and talents? The participants were given two additional weeks to complete this assignment with a 20-photo maximum. The same procedures from the initial assignment were used during individual meetings with participants to discuss their second assignment photos with only minimal revision to the probing questions to reflect the differences in assignments.

Upon completion of these interviews, programme staff once again conducted a debriefing meeting to discuss similarities, differences and themes across participants' photos. Using the two assignments, six primary themes were identified that were consistent across the participants. One photograph was selected to represent each of the primary themes, being careful to ensure that each photographer was represented in this final selection (two participants' photos were used to jointly illustrate one theme resulting in six themes across the seven photographers). The resulting seven photographs and six themes were used to lead a group discussion with the participants.

Phase two progressed to a group discussion where each participant was asked to explain his/her photo to the entire group of participants. Then all of the participants were encouraged to respond to the photo and theme. This group discussion also served as a member check in order for researchers to verify the relevance of the identified themes and whether the themes were 'true for them' (i.e., representative of the group as a whole). It also provided an opportunity for the participants to further elaborate on their perspectives and what they wanted the community to know about these themes. Programme staff conducted a final debriefing session to review the information gathered during the group meeting. Programme staff were unanimous in agreement that the identified themes had been validated by the group discussion and proceeded to identify quotes that best illustrated participant perspectives in their own voice.

Phase three

Phase three consisted of final preparations for two community exhibitions: a pilot exhibition at the local Arc and a primary exhibition at a community location. The exhibitions consisted of one large group display, as well as individual displays for each photographer. The large group display included one enlarged (i.e., 54 cm × 74 cm), framed picture from each of the participants representing one of the six prominent themes. Each photograph was accompanied by a narrative that described the theme using quotes from the group discussion and individual meetings to reflect the 'voice' of the group. In addition, each photographer had an individual display that consisted of one poster collage containing five photos that represented the participant, one 'My Story' photo book containing all of the photos the participant had taken and props that related to the participant's displayed ideas (e.g., fishing pole for a participant who was a knowledgeable fisherman). Individual poster collages were also accompanied by narratives using quotes from the individual interviews. Additionally, participants stood by their displays during the exhibitions so that attendees could ask them any questions about their photographs and experiences in the Photovoice project.

The participants were also encouraged to invite their friends and families to the pilot exhibition that was held at the local Arc headquarters. The purpose of this exhibition was to provide a venue for participants to display their findings to their friends and family in a comfortable and familiar environment, and to practise speaking to others about the meanings of their photographs. The pilot exhibition provided an opportunity to experiment with the display in order to make the necessary adjustments for the primary exhibition. Once the pilot exhibition ended, preparation for the primary exhibition focused on marketing so as to create maximum community impact. It was beneficial and necessary to invite key members of the community who represented a broad variety of constituents. Held at the city's Chamber of Commerce located in the downtown area, the primary exhibition attendees included an invitation list consisting of friends and family members of the photographers, local policy-makers, service providers, government representatives and general citizens.

Data collection and analysis

Research question #1: photographer perceptions

This research was approved by the university's Institutional Review Board and all participants provided informed consent for the collection of data prior to the programme. Photographs taken by participants were collected as the primary data-set. Digital images were downloaded from participants' cameras to portable hard drives (for secure data storage purposes) and viewed on laptop computers during the individual interviews. Individual interviews and the group discussion were digitally audio-recorded. Interviews ranged from 60 to 90 minutes, and the group discussion was 90 minutes in length. All digital audio-recordings were transcribed verbatim, and participant photographs were systematically assigned numbers. During individual interviews and group discussion, these assigned numbers were referenced in order for the statements to be linked to the photographs under discussion. This documentation procedure enabled the researchers to examine photographs as well as the accompanying statements from the transcripts during data analysis.

A constant comparative approach (Patton 2002) was taken to data analysis. After interviews had been completed with each participant, programme staff met to discuss the content of pictures and transcripts. Through the discussion, arising themes were identified. Identified themes were then discussed in relation to each participant and across participants to ensure that they were truly representative and to explore alternative explanations. This systematic approach was used until consensus was reached regarding the dimensions of the identified themes. Individual interview transcripts were then systematically coded using the identified themes and reviewed again by the researchers to ensure that they were consistent within and across participants and that all primary concepts had been captured.

As described earlier, six prominent themes were identified by programme staff during the debriefing meetings. These themes were presented to the Photovoice participants at the group discussion as a member check (Jurkowski 2008; Patton 2002), where their accuracy and relevance were validated and the meaning of themes was further expounded upon by the participants. Based on this validation, the transcript of the group discussion was coded using the same system that was implemented for the individual interviews. This allowed for easy retrieval of coded statements representative of the identified themes. Narratives that accompanied photographs in the exhibitions were developed and based on thematic coding using the prominent themes of all the Photovoice data.

Research question #2: community outcomes

Attendees of the primary Photovoice community exhibition were asked to complete an anonymous survey upon exiting. The survey consisted of a demographic question regarding the respondent's role in the community, six Likert scale questions and two open-ended questions. The survey collected information regarding their perceptions of the exhibition and the issues which were identified, how it impacted them personally, if they planned to take any actions based on their experience and the community's capacity to address the issues that surfaced. Descriptive analyses (i.e. frequencies, means and standard deviations) were conducted on the data collected from the exhibition attendees. Due to the small sample size and limited variance in subject's respective roles in the community, it was not possible to conduct one-way analysis of variance to assess whether community outcomes differed significantly by community role.

Results

The two research questions that were used to address the photographers' perspectives on their own place and inclusion within the community, and any impacts that these photos and narratives had on a community generated many ideas. It was revealed that the participants had many strengths and talents that, if recognized, would be valued in the community. Additionally, these photographers had a strong desire to be connected to others and to their larger communities however this was defined. Many wished to live independently and be gainfully employed. That said, several individuals spoke about their loneliness, hurt feelings and a sense of being dependent on their family members and church for their social connections and to gain a sense of their own importance.

Perceptions on community access, participation and inclusion

Specifically, six themes were identified and included: (a) a desire for community membership and to achieve a sense of belonging, (b) a desire for independence and to live independently, (c) having talents and abilities to share that were not readily recognized by the community, (d) consumerism and a sense of independence and opportunities for choice that were associated with the earning of money, (e) a desire to be treated as adults and (f) limited connections to and opportunities in the community. We decided to expound upon the results of the first two themes (i.e. community membership and desire for independence) as the participants' needs to belong and live actively in the community appear to be the most relevant themes that were associated with an improved quality of life and greater self-determination. However, the remaining four themes are supportive of these two prominent ones and will be discussed within that context.

A desire for community membership and a sense of belonging

The participants explained how simple it was to be made to feel welcomed, including such common courtesies as, 'being friendly, smiling and speaking to me'; 'asking me my name'; 'knowing my name'; and 'when you ask them something, they are willing to help'. Patrick emphasized that 'The one thing that comes to mind is being respected'. When asked to elaborate on what this meant, he stated, 'Respect is having friends who actually say "I'm glad you're here. I hope you have a great time"'. Feeling unwelcomed was associated with a lack of basic courtesy on the part of others, such as 'They walk away when you speak to them', and 'They don't listen to me'. Garrett also stated, 'Sometimes when you go to a place you don't know, you have mixed feelings . . . they don't want to help you'. Church was mentioned by several participants as a place where they felt welcomed. Lisa remarked that 'I feel welcomed at church because every Sunday we have to get up and shake everybody's hand'.

The participants identified few other places where they truly felt welcomed and accepted, except for family and church events. These limited community connections, another recurrent theme revealed in this research, were apparently reinforced by the unwelcomed feelings described above. There is a hesitancy to step out of the comfortable, familiar relationships provided by family and church. However, Garrett found a sense of belonging connected with his place of employment. He had worked in the dining hall of a university campus for the past 15 years. Even though his job did not begin until 4 pm in the afternoon, he arrived on campus three hours prior, not out of necessity but because he liked to arrive early. Pointing to a photo he took on campus, he proclaimed, 'It's the Elliott Center. That is where I spend half of my day'. He stated that he used the extra time before work to go to the library to check his email, visit the food court, socialize with friends and sometimes visit the shops near to the campus. He felt secure on the campus, 'Because I have friends that work on campus'. Having friends that worked there had increased his sense of belonging which was supported by his statement, 'It makes me feel important'. He also noted the importance of feeling independent on campus. In addition to several faculty and staff members, he knew a number of students. He proudly noted that 'Some of the students know me through class, from presenting in class. We talk every once in a while'. The fact that 'They know me without my [university work] name tag on' really seemed to boost his sense of belonging and feeling connected to students and staff alike.

Similar stories were not forthcoming from the other photographers. There were even times when Garrett felt excluded. He described seeing activities occurring on campus in which he would like to take part but did not. He stated that 'We [people with disabilities] feel sheltered sometimes. The public does not welcome many people with disability. And I am afraid that I couldn't do it'. When asked what someone might say if he were to try to participate, he stated that 'They will say look at that handicapped person'. When asked, 'So you just don't even want to try'? he replied, 'Right'. However, he knew exactly what it would take for him to feel more comfortable participating, 'Yeah if I could . . . an instructor could come up to you and show you. Like if you had a one-on-one to show how and go over the steps with you'.

Yet, even when skills were apparent to family and church members, there was a disconnect in using these skills to access the greater community. Typically, people use their talents and skills to access venues for connecting with others (Anderson and Kress 2003). However, these photographers had limited opportunities to share their strengths. For example, David was an avid fisherman and had developed significant skill in this pursuit. He readily explained how he managed multiple reels at once, stating, 'See, I have one [rod] in my hand, and three out there waiting for a fish'. When asked who knew about his fishing skills and knowledge, he replied that he only went fishing with his family. The lack of community participation and inclusion precluded the sharing of these talents with others, and their talents were not being used as tools to connect to the community in social ways.

A desire for independence and to live independently

One particular photo stood out to the project staff, but not for the reason that was intended by the photographer. The photographer, William, was a student in a post-secondary education programme associated with the local university and lived in a student apartment complex near the campus. William's focus was on his prized Special Olympics medal, which he had displayed on his desk in his apartment among a pile of papers and dirty dishes. Photovoice staff, however, noted how much the photo reminded them of their college days and the newfound independence that comes with not always having to clean your dishes and being able to do what you want in your own apartment. When asked if he got into trouble for not cleaning his dishes and putting them away, he stated proudly and with a great deal of satisfaction, 'Nope'! This photographer proceeded to share with the other participants, all of whom lived with their parents, what independence felt like. William declared:

> I'm living on my own and it's just a great life for me. When I'm there [campus housing], I have freedom and I get out in the community and make friends, meet new people, and it's just been a great life for me . . . living with your parents, they tell you what to do, and living on your own, you don't have all that, so it's a great life.

Perhaps more telling than this young man's words was the smile that was clearly evident as he spoke of his independent living situation.

In addition to their desire for independence, photographers shared a parallel theme of a desire to be treated as an adult, rather than continuing to be regarded as a dependent child. Feelings of embarrassment were discussed, including comments such as 'it hurts your feelings', 'being picked on is one of my biggest things', and 'you don't feel comfortable', with specific examples of being offered children's menus in restaurants and questions being posed to accompanying adults, rather than directed to the individual with a disability. Participants expressed frustration with the general public who frequently treated them as if they were children. Patrick summed up the group's sentiments by stating, 'You should treat us the way we are. We are adults. We're not kids'.

When the other photographers were asked if they ever thought about living on their own, there were several affirmative responses such as 'in the future' and 'I think about it'. In fact, when asked if they would like to live on their own, all participants responded in the affirmative. However, there was also some noticeable apprehension, as Taylor admitted:

> I've talked to Mom and Dad about it . . . I told them I wish I could be on my own; to be independent and on my own. But I have to live with my parents. It would be better for me. I can't live on my own. I can't do it.

The one exception was a photographer who had previously admitted that he paid for room and board. Patrick's pictures included depictions of himself helping out with household chores. He stated:

> I'd like to one day own a house, where I can do the dishes, the laundry, the cooking and the cleaning, all of that. I just love to do it . . . It makes me who I am; a person who is more independent.

Yet, even Patrick could not identify a clear plan for establishing his independent living scenario. There was also some apprehension about what the future held since most were not living independently. For example, one participant asked, 'What's out there for us, say if our parents are gone in the future'?

Nonetheless, the pride associated with paying your own way and preparing for the responsibility of maintaining a household was evident and was closely tied with being treated as an adult who is gainfully employed and has the rights of any consumer in the community. Discussions revealed that consumerism was highly valued by all of the photographers, who expressed their need, and indeed their right, to make choices and purchases with their well-earned money. For example, Taylor said of his purchasing power, 'I work really hard for that money. I deserve it'. Lisa equated the opportunity to use her own money with her independence and stated, 'I pay for the movie ticket with my own money. I like to be independent; on my own'.

Community outcomes

The primary Photovoice exhibition was attended by 122 community members, while the exit survey was completed by 74 attendees. The majority of respondents to the exit survey were family members and friends of the Photovoice participants (48%). The remaining attendees were general community members (24%), university students and faculty (23%), and service providers to individuals with disabilities (5%).

Attendees overwhelmingly provided positive feedback about the exhibition (see Table 3 for a presentation of findings from the exit survey). This may not be a surprising finding given the large percentage of respondents who were family members or friends of the participants. All respondents found that attending the exhibition was a valuable investment of their time and they felt that it had positively impacted on their perceptions of individuals with intellectual disabilities. All but 3% felt that the exhibition increased their awareness of issues concerning community participation and inclusion. Although attendees were confident in the community's capacity to address the main issues identified at the exhibition (i.e. 72% strongly agree, 28% agree), they had somewhat less confidence in their own abilities to address these issues (i.e. 53% strongly agree, 44% agree).

Two open-ended questions were asked on the exit survey: (1) which photo and caption did you learn the most from or find the most interesting? Why? And (2) is

Table 3. Photovoice exhibition attendees' perceptions of their experience.

Variable	N	m	sd
Valuable investment of my time	74	3.81	0.394
Increased my awareness of issues	74	3.73	0.505
Changed my understanding of the issues	73	3.66	0.506
There are things I (or my organization) can begin to do to address the issues	68	3.47	0.657
Positively impacted my perceptions of people with intellectual disabilities	73	3.79	0.407
Community has the capacity to address the issues	72	3.72	0.451

Note: Likert scale: 1 = strongly disagree, 2 = disagree, 3 = agree, 4 = strongly agree.

there anything else that you would like to share with us about the Photovoice exhibition and this experience? Responses to the first question demonstrated that all of the primary photos and narratives presented at the exhibition had a strong impact on attendees' understanding of the issues the photographers wished to communicate to the community. Attendees had obviously taken the time to read the narratives accompanying the photographs and process their meaning. Responses included statements such as:

> The photo of the mailbox – waiting for the mail every single day as a highlight was pretty powerful. The photo of one photographer eating pizza and drinking a beer as it relates to being treated as an adult. The photo of church and the caption that many individuals had strong connections with church (e.g. shaking hands at church really makes them feel welcomed). The photos of the photographers as consumers who have money to spend.

> No specific one . . . but reading the narratives greatly expanded my understanding of some of the issues these people face and also ways that I can better relate!
> The views of the participants plus their accomplishments – that they know they are adults, that life has difficulties and that they want to be taken seriously.

Responses to the second open-ended question were overwhelmingly positive, and many found it to be a 'powerful learning experience'. As one individual stated, 'This was a much needed experience for the participants and for those who came to view their work. They all have a voice that needs to be heard'. However, visitors to the exhibition also noted that there was a need to attract additional attendees (e.g. 'Get more people out here so that people can be exposed to these issues') and to display the pictures and narratives in different locations (e.g. 'Spread these photos and captions for local companies to exhibit;' 'The more they are seen, the more people will understand and enjoy!;' and 'More venues for people to see this excellent exhibit').

Discussion

Through Photovoice we observed a cohort of adults with myriad talents, skills and gifts. Gardeners, choir singers, expert fishermen and competent photographers were noted among the group. Nevertheless, we observed and heard reports of minimal access and limited acceptance in recreational, physical and social activity pro-grammes. Participants reported being ignored and patronized, and rarely felt welcomed to join programmes of their own choice as active members. Social isolation was a significant concern, since access to peers and activities had not been effective components of their school, post-school or vocational programmes. Although a majority of the participants were employed, they typically only worked 6 to 8 hours per week. A report of substantial amounts of discretionary time with little to do was the norm. Consequently, individuals frequently experienced anxiety, boredom and loneliness due to the social isolation and abundance of free time they had, despite their desire to be active members of their community. The social isolation experienced by this group of adults with ID/DD was consistent with that described in the literature (e.g. Carter et al. 2012; National Disability Rights Network 2011; Zijlstra and Vlaskamp 2005).

Our findings have implications for the self-advocacy movement, the local community and the sharing of responsibility for inclusion, as well as future research using Photovoice with individuals with ID/DD and the research questions that we need to be studying in the future. Self-advocates must be the experts regarding their own lives, as nobody understands their needs or sees the obstacles to their access, as well as they themselves do. It should be left up to these individuals to help determine which issues and plans have currency within the broader community. With a voice, self-advocates help communities identify practices and solutions to overcome what was once considered to be unsolvable.

It was evident from the research that participants were socially isolated, lonely and lack (i.e. but desire) greater community access and membership. While exhibition attendees felt that the community had the capacity to address these issues, their lack of confidence in their own abilities to assist with this effort demonstrated a potential disconnect with the meaning of 'community'. Perhaps attendees' perceptions of a community as they relate to individuals with intellectual disabilities are of the compulsory provision of government services that support these individuals. Rather, it should be a collection of residents, such as themselves, who share a collective responsibility for the quality of life of all of their neighbours. It will be the responsibility of the entire Photovoice team, including self-advocates, to secure additional locations to display the photos and the accompanying narratives across the community to further the impact on the local community. In addition, the research team will continue to work with Photovoice participants to identify and take advocacy steps to increase their social inclusion and community participation.

Conclusions

There are limitations to the presented study that should be considered. Firstly, the findings are representative of a small group of individuals with ID/DD from a southeastern US community with a population of nearly 300,000 people. There may be limited generalizability beyond these individuals and their community.

Secondly, the potential influences of both participants' assistants and project staff must be acknowledged. Great effort was put into mitigating these types of influences by clearly delineating the roles of assistants from those of participants, continually reminding participants that it was their voice that needed to be heard, redirecting interviews back to participants if assistants stepped in unnecessarily and empowering participants to disagree and communicate their own points of view (e.g. a programme staff member responding to a participant in the group discussion who shook his head 'no' by stating, 'Sam, I noticed you shook your head "no", and I'm glad you did that because we don't all have to agree. Can you tell us how you feel'?).

However, individuals with ID/DD are sometimes easily influenced in a desire to please others (Snell et al. 2009), and comments made by assistants and staff members may have unintentionally impacted participants.

Thirdly, the majority of respondents to the primary exhibition exit survey were family members and friends of the participants. Therefore, we gained little perspective on how the Photovoice exhibition impacted community perspectives on the inclusion of individuals with ID/DD. Despite these limitations, we believe the findings are still of relevance since they are consistent with the literature, yet expand upon our understanding of community access, participation and inclusion, as they directly represent the perspectives of individuals with ID/DD in their own voices.

Few adults with ID/DD have had sufficient experiences to influence the very communities in which they live and to improve their quality of life. This is because they generally lack the skills and opportunities to make choices (Brown and Brown 2009), have low self-esteem, lack assertiveness skills and the communities in which they live lack any concern for their welfare (Schleien, Ray and Green 1997). As practitioners, agencies and communities attempt to address problems associated with accessibility to encourage broader participation by under-served populations, and encourage system changes that support inclusive service delivery, it is necessary for these approaches to be undertaken and skills learned by myriad stakeholders. Only with their values and voices clearly heard by others within the community, and at multiple levels of organizations, will underrepresented people, such as those with ID/DD, be empowered to influence their communities and become more self-determined. Only with a voice at the table will they be able to share their perspectives, needs and desires to assist in the redesign of policies and practices that affect their recreation, fitness, socialization, inclusion and personal growth.

In essence, community leaders, recreation practitioners, teachers and citizens must assess the health of their agencies, programmes and activities with assistance from those individuals who are seen to be underrepresented and marginalized. This willingness and ability to listen to and collaborate with these under-served consumers is a far cry from the usual manner in which we typically design experiences, and should help the community better meet the needs of those they wish to serve. The perspectives of individuals with ID/DD are blatantly missing from service delivery, community inclusion and quality of life research. Several researchers argue that the professionally driven research that dominates the literature to date is missing 'the voice' of those who are most impacted by the policies and practices in place, and that there is a need for change (e.g. Aldridge 2007).

The results of this project point to a number of additional research questions that should be addressed so that we may further understand the recreation and social needs, as well as the desire for acceptance and independence, of those who have been excluded from our communities. For example, what are the barriers (or constraints) that individuals with ID/DD perceive to community access and participation; how do they define friendship and other social relationships; and what actions are they taking to gain greater access and become more engaged in the community? Moreover, how does Photovoice contribute to preparing individuals with ID/DD to be competent and influential self-advocates and community leaders? This also points to the need to complete the Photovoice process with additional stakeholders. For example, how do parents and other caregivers of persons with ID/DD perceive their sons' and daughters' community preferences, access and participation, and what do recreation and park professionals see as the barriers and supports to including this population in their programme offerings?

The field and society in general have come a long way in making recreation programmes more available and communities more accessible to people with ID/DD. However, agencies must go much further by actively recruiting and encouraging their participation through the shaping of service delivery so as to provide opportunities to articulate their opinions, concerns and desires. Perhaps self-advocacy tools such as Photovoice will help fill this void by empowering all parties to get a better handle on individuals' needs and wishes to become more engaged and gain greater access to the community. If family members, advocates, service providers, researchers and policy-makers continue to listen to the preferences and dreams of people with disabilities, and to build on their abilities and contributions, and if we cultivate the development of community groups that are truly open to diverse ideas, people with ID/DD will prosper in areas of the community that formerly appeared to be out of their reach. We believe it is most fitting to conclude with the words of Patrick, one of the Photovoice participants: 'We all have a voice. What we say with that voice, we show through our pictures'.

Funding

The development and dissemination of this manuscript was partially supported by Cooperative Agreement No. H325K070330 funded by the Office of Special Education Programs, Office of Special Education and Rehabilitative Services, US Department of Education.

Conflict of interest

The content and opinions expressed herein do not necessarily reflect the position or policy of the US Department of Education, and no official endorsement should be inferred.

Notes on contributors

Stuart J. Schleien, Ph.D., is Professor and Chair of the Department of Community and Therapeutic Recreation at the University of North Carolina at Greensboro (UNCG). As a Licensed and Certified Therapeutic Recreation Specialist, he has developed best practices that have helped parents and professionals design inclusive community services.

Lindsey Brake is a Student Life Advisor, focusing on inclusion with Beyond Academics at UNCG. Ms. Brake's professional background is in therapeutic recreation and community inclusion.

Kimberly D. Miller, MS, CPRP is an AP Assistant Professor and Research Associate in the Department of Community and Therapeutic Recreation at UNCG. Her research interests have focused on the inclusion of individuals with intellectual and developmental disabilities in the community.

Ginger Walton is the Community Resource Specialist for The Arc of Greensboro. Ms. Walton's professional background is in clinical nursing, where as a family nurse practitioner she provided developmental assessments, education, and guidance for families.

References

Aldridge, J. 2007. "Picture This: The Use of Participatory Photographic Research Methods with People with Learning Disabilities." *Disability and Society* 22 (1): 1–17. doi:10.1080/09687590601056006.

Anderson, L., and C. B. Kress. 2003. *Inclusion: Including People with Disabilities in Parks and Recreation Opportunities.* State College, PA: Venture

Booth, T., and W. Booth. 2003. "In the Frame: Photovoice and Mothers with Learning Difficulties." *Disability & Society* 18 (4): 431–442. doi:10.1080/0968759032000080986.

Brown, I., and R. I. Brown. 2009. "Choice as an Aspect of Quality of Life for People with Intellectual Disabilities." *Journal of Policy and Practice in Intellectual Disabilities* 6 (1): 11–18. doi:10.1111/j.1741-1130.2008.00198.x.

Carter, E., B. Swedeen, M. C. M. Walter, and C. K. Moss. 2012. "'I Don't Have to Do This by Myself?' Parent-Led Community Conversations to Promote Inclusion." *Research & Practice for Persons with Severe Disabilities* 37 (1): 9–23. doi:10.2511/027494812800903184.

Clement, T., and C. Bigby. 2009. "Breaking Out of a Distinct Social Space: Reflections of Supporting Community Participation for People with Severe and Profound Intellectual Disability." *Journal of Applied Research in Intellectual Disabilities* 22 (3): 264–275. doi:10.1111/j.1468-3148.2008.00458.x.

Devine, M. A., and B. King. 2006. "Research Update: The Inclusion Landscape." *Parks and Recreation* 41 (5): 22–25.

Frieri, P. 1973. *Education for Critical Consciousness.* New York: Seabury Press.

Horwitz, S., B. Kerker, P. Owens, and E. Zigler. 2000. *The Health Status and Needs of People with Mental Retardation.* New Haven, CT: School of Medicine and Special Olympics, Yale University.

Jurkowski, J. M. 2008. "Photovoice as Participatory Action Research Tool for Engaging People with Intellectual Disabilities in Research and Program Development." *Intellectual and Developmental Disabilities* 46 (1): 1–11. doi:10.1352/0047-6765(2008)46[1:PAPART]2.0.CO;2.

Jurkowski, J., and A. Paul-Ward. 2007. "Photovoice with Vulnerable Populations: Addressing Disparities in Health Promotion among People with Intellectual Disabilities." *Health Promotion Practice* 8 (4): 358–365. doi:10.1177/1524839906292181.

Jurkowski, J., Y. Rivera, and J. Hammel. 2009. "Health Perceptions of Latinos with Intellectual Disabilities: The Results of a Qualitative Pilot Study." *Health Promotion Practice* 10 (1): 144–155. doi:10.1177/1524839907309045.

Killion, C. M., and C. C. Wang. 2000. "Linking African American Mothers across Life Stage and Station through Photovoice." *Journal of Health Care for the Poor and Underserved* 11 (3): 310–325. doi:10.1353/hpu.2010.0816.

Miller, K. D., S. J. Schleien, and J. Lausier. 2009. "Search for Best Practices in Inclusive Recreation: Programmatic Findings." *Therapeutic Recreation Journal* 43 (1): 27–41. doi:10.1177/1524839907309045.

National Disability Rights Network. 2011. *A Call to Action! The Future of the Disability Service System to Provide Quality Work.* Washington, DC: National Disability Rights Network.

Paiewonsky, M. 2011. "Hitting the Reset Button on Education: Student Reports on Going to College." *Career Development for Exceptional Individuals* 34 (1): 31–44. doi:10.1177/0885728811399277.

Patton, M. Q. 2002. *Qualitative Research & Evaluation Methods.* 3rd ed. Thousand Oaks, CA: Sage.

Poudrier, J., and R. T. Mac-Lean. 2009. "'We've Fallen into the Cracks': Aboriginal Women's Experiences with Breast Cancer through Photovoice." *Nursing Inquiry* 16 (4): 306–317. doi:10.1111/j.1440-1800.2009.00435.x.

Sable, J. R., and J. Gravink. 2005. "The PATH to Community Health Care of People with Disabilities: A Community-based Therapeutic Recreation Service." *Therapeutic Recreation Journal* 39 (1): 78–87.

Schleien, S., K. Miller, and M. Shea. 2009. "Search for Best Practices in Inclusive Recreation: Preliminary Findings." *Journal of Park and Recreation Administration* 27 (1): 17–34.

Schleien, S. J., M. T. Ray, and F. P. Green. 1997. *Community Recreation and People with Disabilities: Strategies for Inclusion.* 2nd ed. Baltimore: Paul H. Brookes.

Snell, M. E., R. Luckasson, S. Borthwick-Duffy, V. Bradley, W. H. E. Buntinx, D. L. Coulter, E. P. Craig, et al. 2009. "Characteristics and Needs of People with Intellectual Disability Who Have Higher IQ's." *Intellectual and Developmental Disabilities* 47 (3): 220–233. doi:10.1352/1934-9556-47.3.220.

Wang, C., and M. A. Burris. 1994. "Empowerment through Photo-novella: Portraits of Participation." *Health Education and Behavior* 21 (2): 171–186. doi:10.1177/109019819402100204.

Wang, C., and M. A. Burris. 1997. "Photovoice: Concept, Methodology, and Use for Participatory Needs Assessment." *Health Education and Behavior* 24 (3): 369–387.

Wang, C. C., J. Cash, and L. Power. 2000. "Who Knows the Streets as Well as the Homeless? Promoting Personal and Community Action through Photovoice." *Health Promotion Practice* 1 (1): 81–89.

Zijlstra, H. P., and C. Vlaskamp. 2005. "Leisure Provision for Persons with Profound Intellectual and Multiple Disabilities: Quality Time or Killing Time?" *Journal of Intellectual Disability Research* 49 (6): 434–448.

The relationship among motivational environment, autonomous self-regulation and personal variables in refugee youth: implications for mental health and youth leadership

Kiboum Kim[a], David M. Compton[b] and Bryan McCormick[a]

[a]*Department of Recreation, Park & Tourism Studies, Indiana University, Bloomington, IN, USA;*
[b]*Department of Environmental Health, Indiana University, Bloomington, IN, USA*

This study examined the influence of motivational conditions and personal variables of refugee youth on self-regulation to perform roles in a leadership programme designed for refugee youth. Eighteen refugee youth participated in this study, selected from those previously engaged in a pilot study (veterans, $n = 4$) and those newly recruited (novices, $n = 14$). Data for self-regulation were collected using the Situational Self-Regulation Questionnaire for Participation. Hierarchical linear modelling was utilized to test the study hypotheses. Results indicated that three personal variables including gender, experience in an autonomy-supportive environment and interaction effects between these two variables explained 37% of variance between participants in self-regulation. Furthermore, the type of motivational environment was a significant indicator, explaining the level of self-regulation. Participants in an autonomous-supportive environment reported 3.84 units higher self-regulation than those in a controlled environment ($\beta_{01} = -3.84$, $t = -3.30$, df $= 18$, $p < 0.01$). However, there was no interaction effect between variables and the type of motivational environment.

Introduction

Exhibiting autonomous motivation for youth is critical for successful participation in social, cultural, leisure, civic and educational aspects of life because of its pivotal role in human development. There is compelling evidence that autonomous motivation leads to greater task engagement (Connell and Wellborn 1991; Assor, Kaplan, and Roth 2002), greater persistence (Pelletier et al. 2001; Ryan and Deci 2007), greater satisfaction (Deci et al. 1981; Ryan and Grolnick 1986) and higher task performance (Ryan and Deci 2007; Standage, Duda, and Ntoumanis 2005) compared to controlled motivation or amotivation. These facets of human development are not only important for all youth but also essential to recently resettled refugee youth who are struggling to become a part of the new culture. However, the capacity for autonomy among refugee youth relocated to host countries appears problematic.

According to the United Nations High Commissioner for Refugees (UNHCR 2011a), less than 1% out of 15.4 million refugees are placed in resettlement countries annually including the USA, Canada and Australia. The USA is the leading resettlement county, hosting more than half of newly resettled refugees. More than 72,000 refugee youth under age of 18 were admitted to the USA between 2008 and

2010 (United States Department of Homeland Security 2011). Prior to residing in the USA, many refugee youth experienced traumatic events in their homeland and refugee camps such as witnessing torture and death, separation from family members and deprivation of basic human needs (Harrell-Bond 2000; Murray et al. 2008; Pynoos, Kinzie, and Gordon 2001). These traumatic events resulted in high rates of mental illness including depression, anxiety and post-traumatic stress disorder (PTSD) (Derluyn and Broekaert 2007; WHO 2005). Furthermore, refugee youth exhibit diminished self-esteem and self-efficacy, as well as learned helplessness as a consequence of experiences in refugee camps where they were deprived of basic human rights and had to fend for their survival (Kirk and Cassity 2007). The opportunity for refugee youth to make autonomous choices appears to be deprived after resettlement due to a lack of social, parental and financial support, as well as long-standing ethnic, religious and cultural beliefs (Mackenzie, McDowell, and Pittaway 2007).

While recovering from displacement, relocation and abhorrent living conditions, refugee youth are asked to perform the same daily tasks as youth currently living in the USA such as school work, peer interaction, personal care and self-development. In addition, they are expected to execute a number of parental delegated or assigned tasks required for successful resettlement and acculturation (Liebkind, Jasinskaja-Lahti, and Solheim 2004; Zhou 2001). Success in performing these tasks may accelerate adjustment to resettlement while failure is associated with high rates of school dropout, engagement in antisocial behaviours, delayed socialization, acculturation stress and difficulty in securing employment (Birman and Trickett 2001; Derluyn and Broekaert 2007; Loughry and Flouri 2001).

Unlike youth in the USA, the opportunity to experience autonomous choices was rare for refugee youth due to threatening living conditions in their homeland (Lustig et al. 2004; Mackenzie, McDowell, and Pittaway 2007) and years of living in refugee camps where their freedoms are often controlled by the host government (Yoshikawa 2005). In addition, placing refugee youth under daily conditions where they are expected to assume adult roles can result in the restriction of the potential for autonomous choices in their lives. Constraining or prohibiting autonomous motivation in refugee youth may suppress independence, hamper upwards mobility and lead to continued marginalization of refugees (UNHCR 2011b). In this context, providing refugee youth with opportunities to increase their capacity for autonomy to perform ascribed or acquired leadership roles (e.g. effective speakers, translator, mediator, decision maker and risk manager) may be essential to execute challenging tasks required for successful adjustment during the immediate resettlement process and in the future (Gale 2011).

Literature review
Refugee youth and mental health

The Immigration and Nationality Act (United States Citizenship and Immigration Services 2008) defines a refugee population as 'aliens who are unable or unwilling to return to their countries of origin or nationality because of persecution or a well-founded fear of persecution'. According to the United States Department of Homeland Security, more than 200,000 refugees were admitted into the USA between 2008 and 2010 (United States Department of Homeland Security 2011).

Refugees to the USA represent over 70% of the more than 80,000 refugees who are resettled globally each year (UNCHR 2011a). Refugee youth come from a number of different countries bringing with them unique experiences as they seek to adjust to life in America. Lustig et al. (2004) characterized their experiences in the three stages of (1) preflight, (2) flight and (3) resettlement.

The preflight phase refers to the period of time living in their country of origin. A number of exploratory studies (e.g., Harrell-Bond 2000; Khanlou et al. 2002; Zabaneh, Watt, and O'Donnell 2008) reporting experiences in refugee youth have described the relentless realities of war, famine, and political and religious persecution. As a result of these experiences, a significant number of refugee youth exhibit mental disorders including symptoms of anxiety and depression, relationship and behavioural problems (Derluyn and Broekaert 2007; Hjern, Angel, and Hoejer 1991), and PTSD (Allwood, Bell-Dolan, and Husain 2002; Henley and Robinson 2011). Lifetime prevalence rates for PSTD among refugee youth have been found to be two to four times higher than for non-traumatized groups living in the USA (WHO 2005). Evidence indicates that individuals suffering from symptoms of PTSD demonstrate lower levels of autonomy (Kolts, Robinson, and Tracy 2004; Sato and McCann 1997) as well as decreased self-esteem and self-efficacy (Lustig et al. 2004; Loughry and Flouri 2001). Steele, van der Hart, and Nijenhuis (2001) posit that individuals who are unable to adapt to traumatic experiences subsequently become more dependent, passive and inactive.

The flight phase encompasses the period in refugee camps or in transit to safe places before gaining asylum status in a host country. However, refugee youth frequently endure years of extreme living conditions in relocation camps where access to water, food and medical care, and educational opportunities are limited (Kirk and Cassity 2007). For example, Sommers (2002) concluded that the incidence of acute malnutrition among toddlers living in nine different refugee camps located in Kenya ranged from 20 to 70%. Refugee camps are also closely associated with a high incidence of infectious diseases which can result in serious and consequential impacts on physical development and academic performance (Zabaneh, Watt, and O'Donnell 2008; Tiltnes 2005). In addition, traumatic exposure to violence is often the norm while staying in refugee camps (UNCHR 2011b).

Although a refugee camp provides basic necessities for survival, opportunities for autonomy among the refugees are negligible and almost always compromised. For example, refugees in Thailand are forced to stay in a predetermined territory partitioned with barbed wire fences in order to prevent refugees from coming into contact with the local population (Yoshikawa 2005). They are also forced to become reliant upon assistance from humanitarian agencies while residing in the refugee or detention camps (Mackenzie, McDowell, and Pittaway 2007; Thomas and van Mierop 2004). Additionally, there is frequently little opportunity for empowerment and autonomy or it is strictly controlled or even prohibited by the local or national authorities (Kirk and Cassity 2007; Papadopoulos 2001).

Peterson, Maier, and Seligman (1993) argue that individuals experiencing these conditions where one cannot control events or outcomes tend to exhibit symptoms of learned helplessness which may create generalized expectations for failure in the future. It is notable that individuals identified as experiencing learned helplessness demonstrate low confidence and self-esteem; become passive, inactive and hostile; and blame themselves for their inabilities (Au et al. 2009; Sideridis 2003). Their behaviours are also associated with poor impoverished performance, lack of engagement and weak persistence (Ryan and Deci 2000; Berenson et al. 1997; Gordon and Gordon 2008). During this flight phase refugee youth may be exposed to chaos, unnatural living conditions and a sense of helplessness. As they depart for their new host country, it is apparent that their expectation for resettlement is a better quality of life than during this period.

In the phase of resettlement, refugee youth and their families seek to gain asylum status in a host country. The host country, in most cases, provides only minimal services for resettlement and acculturation such as finding a place to live, looking for a job, enrolling children and youth in a school system and identifying health care services. The resettlement phase provides refugee youth protection from explicit threats such as war, famine or persecution, but at the same time the emigration process can create confusion, challenges and other life stressors associated with navigating new social health and occupational systems (Lustig et al. 2004; Mackenzie, McDowell, and Pittaway 2007; National Child Traumatic Stress Network 2005; Papadopoulos 2001).

For refugee youth, the family and school play important roles in their acculturation, yet they also serve as significant stressors. Since refugee youth tend to assimilate into a new culture better than their parents, it may create conflict between refugee youth and their parents over issues of autonomy, dating and cultural identity (Buki et al. 2003; Kwak 2003). In addition, school can be a risky place for stigmatization associated with ethnicity, religion, insufficient language abilities and socioeconomic status of refugee youth while interacting with their classmates (Liebkind, Jasinskaja-Lahti, and Solheim 2004; Taylor and Turner 2002). Research suggests that refugee youth experience discrimination from their peers in schools and their teachers, have difficulties in building friendships with dominant youth groups and experience heightened stress with academic requirements due to language inadequacies (Wilkinson 2002). The stressors associated with family and peer relationships may result in additional social problems such as high rates of school dropout, teenage pregnancy, reduced social capital and substance abuse (Erath, Flanagan, and Bierman 2007; Jarrett, Sullivan, and Watkins 2005; Lewis et al. 2011).

Overall, both the refugee experience and refugee status in a new host country pose challenges to the mental health of refugee youth. In the refugee process, these youth are repeatedly exposed to traumatic events and environments that erode any perception of autonomy and control, which can lead to passivity, poor self-esteem and expectations for future failure. Once settled in their new host country, the challenges of adaptation and acculturation can further exacerbate these problems.

Challenges facing refugee youth

There are a number of challenges that refugee youth are asked to address while adjusting to their new cultural settings. Many refugee youth are required to assume adult roles earlier than might be expected following resettlement on behalf of their parents or caregivers. For those entering the USA, refugee parents who have limited proficiency in English as well as those who are experiencing difficulties in adjusting to and understanding the new ways of American life may rely more heavily on their children (Birman and Trickett 2001; Derluyn and Broekaert 2007; Weisskirch and Alva 2002). The roles afforded to refugee youth are critical for accelerating social adjustment in most refugee families and societies. However, such role reversal is often a primary cause of conflict within the family and neighbours if refugee youth believe they are forced to perform those roles, rather than being autonomously motivated (Khanlou et al. 2002).

Another challenge among refugee youth is dealing with stressful events in the process of socialization and acculturation such as social rejection, discrimination and prejudice. Continuous experiences of such negative events may result in deteriorating mental health and a delay in social adjustment and engagement. Studies with newly migrated adolescents identified detrimental effects of perceived discrimination on self-efficacy, self-esteem and psychological well-being, as well as academic attainment, interpersonal attitudes, social adjustment, substance use and peer relationships (Foster 2000; Liebkind, Jasinskaja-Lahti, and Solheim 2004; Taylor and Turner 2002). Acculturation stress and stresses associated with displacement are also fairly common among refugees (Lieber et al. 2001; Zhou 2001). The literature is clear in pointing out that building a social network both within and outside of ethnic groups serves as a protective factor (Mesch 2002; Mesch, Turjeman, and Fishman 2008; Oppedal, Roysamb, and Sam 2004).

Acquiring leadership skills is also essential for those refugee youth who suffer from diminished self-values. Studies have indicated that youth in a leadership position demonstrate higher self-esteem, confidence, and social and intellectual competencies (Dimmock and Walker 2000; Lakes 1996; McLaughlin, Irby, and Langman 1994). Studies have also found that children in leadership development programmes show enhanced school performance, positive relationships with peers and successful social adjustment compared to their counterparts (Bloomberg et al. 2003). According to Eccles and Gootman (2002) leadership skills can be nurtured while participating in both academic and non-academic out-of-school activities such as sports, music, religion, and recreation or community services. Refugee youth are recommended to interact with friends in school, during extra-curricular activities, and while in their neighbourhoods. However, there are lower participation rates in extra-curricular activities and community-based activities among refugee youth (Ma and Yeh 2005; Stodolska and Livengood 2006).

Lower participation rates among refugee youth appear to be the product of individual, peer and family factors. Perkins et al. (2007) identified four distinct reasons, including insufficient time, lack of interest in community programmes, negative experience from peers and parental restrictions. Similarly, critical factors facilitating minority youth participation in community-based activities include parental permission, positive models for activity engagement and friends in the activities (Ma and Yeh 2005; Stodolska and Livengood 2006). Additionally, activity fees are a major constraint for ethnic minority youth due to lack of access to funds (Halpern 2002). Of critical importance is ensuring that refugee youth are provided with opportunities to practise and develop leadership skills successfully. Success in leadership acquisition would not only develop refugee youth as potential leaders for their culture and community but also contribute to their personal capacities, mental well-being and potential employment in the future (Fuligni and Hardway 2004; Zeldin and Camino 1999).

Refugee youth and autonomy

Autonomy is a critical issue for refugee youth in order to address challenges discussed previously. However, such factors as lack of social, parental and financial support, as well as long-standing ethnic, religious and cultural beliefs, appear to confound the opportunity for refugee youth to make autonomous choices (Mackenzie, McDowell, and Pittaway 2007). Insufficient household income for refugee families may not allow their children to make an autonomous choice for extra-curricular activities (Yeh et al. 2008). Unlike non-refugee youth raised in the USA where individualism is valued, autonomy for refugee youth immigrating from collectivist cultures is often controlled by their longstanding cultural beliefs and practices (Chakrabarty 2009; Ratner and Hui 2003). In this context, providing refugee youth with opportunities to practise autonomy may be essential to execute challenging tasks required for successful adjustment to, and assimilation in, the American way of life.

Self-determination theory (SDT: Deci and Ryan 1985) suggests that autonomous motivation can be fostered by engaging individuals in an autonomy-supportive environment (ASE). It involves a condition in which an individual can satisfy her/his psychological needs, including competence, autonomy and relatedness (Deci and Ryan 1985; Ryan and Deci 2000). Competence refers to a feeling of capability to succeed in a task. The need for competence can be satisfied when an optimally challenging task is provided with positive and informational feedback. Autonomy is associated with a feeling of choice and control in one's behaviours. It can be promoted by providing choice options, minimizing external controls, offering a meaningful rationale and acknowledging feelings. Finally, the need for relatedness refers to the desire to experience a sense of belonging and connectedness with others (Deci and Ryan 2000; Ryan and Deci 2000). On the other hand, these psychological needs can be thwarted or controlled by external events and agents in a social context, referred to as a controlled environment (Deci and Ryan 1985; Ryan and Deci 2000). Research has found that the need for competence was undermined in conditions in which negative, evaluative and personally controlling feedback were highlighted (Ryan and Deci 2000). Furthermore, an individuals' autonomy appears to be controlled by forcing them to behave in particular ways, emphasizing external reasons for task engagement such as rewards or punishments, and applying threats, pressured evaluations, imposed goals, deadline and surveillance (d'Ailly 2003; Deci and Ryan 2000; Vansteenkiste et al. 2005).

Previous research has attempted to identify techniques that might manipulate the degree of perceived satisfaction in meeting the fundamental psychological needs indicated by SDT. One method, staging techniques, has been effectively utilized in several studies for animating motivational environments (Roark 2008; Rossman and Schlatter 2008; Yost and Ellis 2005). Long et al. (2001) suggested that staging experiences involves manipulating and creating physical and human environments in order for participants to actively involve themselves in the experience and induce intended outcomes. Techniques for staging experiences have been applied in leisure and recreation studies (Ellis, Morris, and Trunnell 1995; Marshall and Ellis 2003; Rossman and Schlatter 2008; Yost and Ellis 2005). For example, a study completed by Long et al. (2001) successfully utilized two programme models as modes of staging experiences. In addition, staging techniques have been utilized in several studies examining the effects of self-determination-based strategies. In a snowshoe tour setting, Yost and Ellis (2005) applied the techniques of staged experiences in order to foster the psychological needs of adolescents. Furthermore, Joussemet et al. (2004) successfully staged four motivational conditions using the presence and absence of rewards and techniques that influence perceived autonomy.

Empirical evidence suggests that autonomous motivation is associated with increased task engagement (Connell and Wellborn 1991; Assor, Kaplan, and Roth 2002); increased persistence (Pelletier et al. 2001; Ryan and Deci 2007); higher task performance (Ntoumanis 2001; Ryan and Deci 2007; Standage, Duda, and Ntoumanis 2005); increased creativity (Amabile, Goldfarb, and Brackfield 1990) and effective problem solving (Black and Deci 2000). On the other hand, students taught with a more controlling approach not only display a lower degree of autonomy but also lose initiative and interest to continue learning (Assor et al. 2005; d'Ailly 2003; Knafo and Assor 2007). As empirical evidence suggests, there are positive outcomes that autonomous motivation contributes to overall well-being in refugee youth. This may bolster refugee youth in accomplishing tasks they may encounter while living in the USA or elsewhere.

The effects of ASE have been examined with different population groups in a variety of study domains including education, health care, religion and physical activity (Hagger, Chatzisarantis, and Biddle 2002; Ryan, Rigby, and King 1993). However, no such study has been conducted with refugee youth. The results of this study may not be consistent with the conclusions of these previous studies. Exhibiting autonomy among refugee youth may require significant time and effort because of diminished self-values due to traumatic experiences in their homeland and refugee camps (Gillespie, Peltzer, and MaClachlan 2000; Lustig et al. 2004). In addition, they may feel uncomfortable while engaging in an autonomous condition because they are familiar with collectivism, long-standing cultural beliefs controlling their autonomy and a situation where tasks are forced upon them to accomplish regardless of their interests, feelings and willingness (Mackenzie, McDowell, and Pittaway 2007; Chakrabarty 2009; Ratner and Hui 2003). For these reasons, the effects of engaging refugee youth in an ASE for the purpose of increasing perceived self-regulation may be delayed or may even not differ from those of youth in a controlling environment. Moreover, the degree of autonomous self-regulation among refugee youth may differ depending on the number of years/months living in the USA or elsewhere. In addition, studies (Amorose and Anderson-Butcher 2007; Amorose and Horn 2000) of self-determination report that levels of autonomy in female groups are significantly higher than those of male groups, while refugee youth studies (Espiritu 1999; Ma and Yeh 2005; Stodolska and Livengood 2006) indicated that female refugee youth are provided with fewer opportunities for autonomous choice than males. Therefore, the purpose of this study is to examine the relationships between autonomous self-regulation, motivational environments (autonomy-supportive vs. controlled) and individual differences among refugee youth while engaging in staged experiences. Three research hypotheses were tested in this study including (1) the variance of self-regulation is significantly explained by participants' variables such as gender, months/years living in the USA and previous autonomous condition experience; (2) the variance of the self-regulation is significantly explained by two types of motivational environments; (3) there is significant interaction effect between the engagement in two motivational environments and participants' variables listed above on increasing self-regulation.

Methods

Study participants

A total of 18 refugee youth participated in this study including fourteen (14) novices and four (4) veterans in terms of whether they had had previous experience as 'Asian Association of Utah Excellence and leadership skills' (AAU EXCELS) Academy members. Eleven participants were male (61.11%) and the mean age was 14.68 years (mode = 15). Participants originated from eight countries including Somalia ($n = 5$), Sudan ($n = 4$), Kenya ($n = 4$), and one of each from Ethiopia, Congo, Ghana, Liberia and Afghanistan. More than half (55.56%) of the study participants had resided in the USA for longer than 53 months (range: 26–71; $\bar{X} = 54$; $\tilde{X} = 53$).

The AAU EXCELS Academy was an extra-curricular activity programme designed for developing leadership skills and demonstrating excellence for refugee youth living in Salt Lake area. The inclusive criteria included (1) 13–16 years of age adolescents; (2) officially classified as 'refugee' status; (3) abilities to read, write and communicate in English; (4) currently enrolled in a middle or senior high school; (5) lived in the USA for two to seven years and (6) no reported juvenile justice violations in the past six months. During the study period, the four veteran members were asked to serve as mentors for the newly recruited participants.

Research design

A 2×2 repeated measures within–between subject design was applied. Two types of staged experiences (controlled environment and ASE) served as the within-subject factor while two groups of study participants (novice and veteran) were considered as a between-subject factor in this study. The repeated measures design was considered as a useful method because the adequate number of data for obtaining high enough statistical power can be gathered by collecting data repeatedly from the small size of participants (Maxwell and Delaney 2004). In addition, a repeated measures design, compared to a between-subject design, was beneficial since the error term caused by individual differences within a group would be ignored because comparisons were made between observations rather than subjects (Maxwell and Delaney 2004).

Measurement

The level of autonomous self-regulation was measured with the Situational Self-Regulation Questionnaire for Participation (SS-ROP) revised from the Exercise Self-Regulation Questionnaire (ES-RQ, Pelletier and Markland 2004). The SS-ROP comprised 12 items which measured the level of four types of motivational orientation including introjected and identified regulation, as well as extrinsic and intrinsic motivation. Each motivational orientation was measured with four items. Participants were asked to read the stem question 'I engage in the group task performance because...' and responded to each item using a 7-point Likert scale ranging from 1 (not at all true) to 7 (very true). Sample items are presented in Table 1. The calculated Cronbach's alphas for each subscale including extrinsic, introjected, identified and intrinsic regulation were 0.81, 0.84, 0.63 and 0.68, respectively.

Table 1. Sample items for each subscale in the SS-RQP.

Subscale	Sample item
Extrinsic motivation	I feel pressured to do it
Introjected regulation	I want others to see me as a good performer
Identified regulation	It is important for self-development
Intrinsic motivation	It will be interesting

Data collection and staged experiences

Equal numbers of novice and veteran participants were randomly assigned into two groups, so that each group consisted of seven novices and two veterans. Data for self-regulation were collected from study participants engaging in experiential activities two times a weekend day over four consecutive weeks (6–27 December 2008). Two experiential activities were introduced to both groups of study participants. Each experiential activity was intentionally animated by trained research staff to create either a controlled environment or an ASE for each group. While one group engaged in a controlled environment, the other group was involved in an ASE where autonomy and perceived competence of the participants might be enhanced. During the second experiential activity, these two groups were engaged using the other treatment condition. The distinct differences between these two treatment conditions were (1) providing several choices versus no choice opportunity in selecting tasks; (2) presenting informational feedback versus evaluative feedback while planning for task completion and (3) focusing on fostering internal perceived locus of causality versus external perceived locus causality.

Three scenario options were prepared for each experiential activity. Each scenario option described a list of tasks required of all group members. Each group assumed at least one of the five selected leadership roles identified from the review of literature in youth leadership including roles such as communicator, decision maker, risk manager, planner and supporter (Aksamit and Rankin 1993; Hesselbein, Goldsmith, and Beckhard 1996). A group in an ASE was asked to choose one from at least three scenario options relying on the group preferences, competence and expected satisfaction rather than tangible benefits (Reeve 2005). After the group selected a scenario, one of the other scenarios was randomly assigned to the other group in a controlled environment. Following this assignment, both groups were allowed 10–20 minutes for planning how to accomplish their scenario tasks. In this process, one trained research staff facilitator was assigned to each group. These facilitators were requested to animate the motivational environment using either a controlled environment or ASE utilizing techniques from studies in self-determination theory (d'Ailly 2003; Deci and Ryan 2000; Yost and Ellis 2005; Vansteenkiste et al. 2005). The techniques utilized by the facilitators are summarized in Table 2.

Immediately following the planning session, participants' perceived autonomy motivation was measured using the SS-RQP. Both groups were asked to perform the assigned or selected scenario by using their group plan. The procedures for data collection and staging experiences are presented in Figure 1. An hour after the participants completed the first staged experience, a second staged experience was provided to both groups. The groups in a controlled environment and an ASE were now engaged in different environmental conditions, respectively. All the other procedures were the same as previously explained.

Data analysis

A Relative Autonomy Index (RAI) for each participant was calculated by creating a weighted sum of the scores using a simple arithmetic. First, the means for each of four regulation types were calculated to form averaged subscale scores. The average scores for all four subscales were then inserted into the following RAI formula:

Table 2. Techniques utilized for animating autonomy-supportive and controlled environments.

Controlled environment	Competence	Autonomous-supportive environment
Provided an evaluative feedback (e.g. 'That is bad idea'), and limited recognition for group efforts (e.g. 'Well done. That was a good plan')	Verbal feedback	Presented informational and positive feedback (e.g., 'I like your idea. If you do, it will be good for preventing potential risks) directly to a specific person (e.g. 'John, you provide a wonderful idea')
Physical feedback was given when participants were asked	Physical feedback	Proposed physical encouragement such as clapping, cheering, asking high five, etc.
N/A	Optimal challenge	Provided possible options with consideration of their abilities for enhancing perceived competence of the group in their planning activity
Controlled environment	*Autonomy*	*Autonomous-supportive environment*
A leadership role was assigned to each member without considering their competence and preference	Choice options	A leadership role was assigned to each member after their opinions and preferences were discussed
Provided a direct solution (e.g. 'You should take this role') using directive expression (should, must or have to), and a direction type of instructions (e.g. 'The first thing that your group has to do is..., and then should do...')	Choice options	Provided possible options if members had a difficulty in making a decision (e.g. 'You may want to explore...'; 'Have you considered other alternatives?')
Promised to provide extrinsic rewards to the group participants	Rationale	Provided a rationale in order to enhance perceived intrinsic locus of causality, integrated motivation and personal values of the experiences
Asked to perform or discharge their responsibilities while completing the assigned group tasks	Acknowledge personal feelings	Participant's feelings were acknowledged (e.g. 'I know it is not an easy task, but...'; 'I understand you are not comfortable in assuming this role, but...')

$RAI = 2(\text{intrinsic extrinsic}) + (\text{identified introjected})$. The RAI score represents the degree of one's perceived feeling of autonomy in a situation (Ryan and Connell 1989).

Two levels of hierarchical linear models with repeated observations nested within participants were utilized to test research hypotheses listed in the previous section (Raudenbush and Bryk 2002). Level-2 statistical variables included (1) months living in the USA (*MLUS*); (2) gender; (3) previous experience (novice vs. veteran) in the AAU EXCELS Academy (*EXP*) and a vector variable representing interaction effects between gender and experience (GenderByEXP). Level-1 variable comprised a grand centred dummy vector representing the effects of two motivational environments ($MoEn_{ti}$–$MoEn$). The dependent variable (Y_{ti}) refers to the self-regulation at observation time t for a participant i. The error term (e_{ti}) represents the residual, which is the amount of deviation between the predicted score and the observed score in self-regulation (Raudenbush and Bryk 2002). Specifically, the model used to test the study hypotheses is presented in Figure 2.

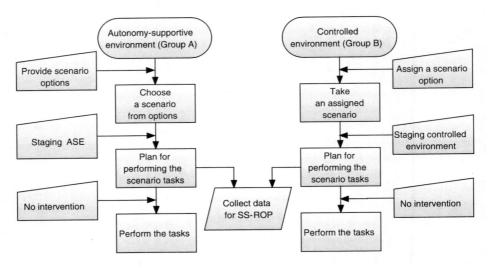

Figure 1. Procedures for data collection and staging experiences.

A null model was tested to determine the significance of the differences in perceived self-regulation associated with variances among participants. An intra-class correlation (ICC) for the null model was calculated and compared with those of alternative models. The first hypothesis was tested using a mean-as-outcome regression technique, which involves constraining the Level-1 coefficient π_{1i} equal to zero while each of the participant-level variables was inserted into the null model. The significances for each of the participants' personal variables were tested (fixed effects). In addition, the variance of random effects explained by the model with Level-2 variables was compared with that of the null model in order to examine how much more variance was explained by the Level-2 variables. The random-coefficient model was considered to test the second hypothesis. This model included the Level-1 variable while the β parameters in Level-2 fixed variables were set to zero. Finally, the last hypothesis was examined through the use of an intercepts- and slopes-as-outcome model. Full model testing of the motivational environment effects on self-regulation among refugee youth was conducted. In order to construct the full model, variables that did not explain more error variance compared to the null model were omitted from the model shown in Figure 2. The variance calculated from the null model was compared with that of full models in order to construct a best fit model explaining self-regulation among refugee youth.

Level 1
$$Y_{ti} = \pi_{0i} + \pi_{1i}(MoEn_{ti} - MoEn..) + e_{ti}$$
Level 2
$$\pi_{0i} = \beta_{00} + \beta_{01}(MLUS) + \beta_{02}(Sex) + \beta_{03}(Exp) + \beta_{04}(SexByExp) + r_{0i}$$
$$\pi_{1i} = \beta_{10} + \beta_{11}(MLUS) + \beta_{12}(Sex) + \beta_{13}(Exp) + \beta_{14}(SexByExp) + r_{1i}$$

for i = 1, 2, ..., *n* persons, where π_{0i} represents the intercept while π_{1i} represents the slopes for participants *i*.

Figure 2. Two levels of hierarchical linear models to test the study hypotheses.

Table 3. Results from the null model.

Fixed effect		Coefficient	SE	t
Intercept (β_{00})		27.62	1.20	23.12*
Random effect	SD	σ^2	df	χ^2
Participants mean (r_{0i})	4.45	19.76	18	73.62*
Level 1 effect (e_{ti})	6.67	44.44		
ICC (ρ) = 0.31				

*$p < 0.001$.

Results

Hypotheses test

The null model was computed to determine if the variation in the self-regulation within and between the study participants existed. The result of the null model revealed that there was significant variation between participants in the levels of self-regulation ($\chi^2 = 73.62$, $p < 0.001$). The ICC was 0.31, indicating that 31% of the variance in self-regulation was between the study participants (Table 3).

This study examined if the variance of self-regulation was significantly explained by participants' variables. The results indicated that the level of self-regulation was significantly associated with the number of months living in the USA ($\beta_{MLUS} = 0.11$, $t = 2.14$, $p < 0.05$) and previous experience ($\beta_{EXP} = 6.49$, $t = 2.78$, $p < 0.05$). Yet, gender of the participant and the interaction effects of gender by experience (GenderByEXP) were not significant at the 0.05 level. The results of variance components analysis showed that the level of self-regulation significantly varied while controlling for the each of the participants' variables. The calculated proportions of variance explained by each of the Level-2 variables (gender, EXP and GenderByEXP) were 0.03, 0.35 and 0.01, respectively. The results of the hypothesis test are presented in Table 4. These three variables in Level-2 were added to the null model. The other variable (MLUS) was excluded because it explained less variance than the null model (Table 5). Approximately, 37% of the true variance between the study participants in self-regulation was additionally accounted for by adding these three Level-2 variables (R^2_{PRE}).

The effect of two types of motivational environments was tested (Table 6). The results indicated that data collected in an ASE showed a higher level of self-regulation than when in a controlled environment ($\beta_{MoEn} = -3.84$, $t = -3.30$, $p < 0.01$). The estimated variance showed that a significant difference existed among the means of the study participants in self-regulation ($\hat{\tau}_{00} = 20.29$, $\chi^2 = 81.49$, df = 18, $p < 0.001$). However, the estimated variance of the slope was not significant ($\hat{\tau}_{11} = 0.85$, $\chi^2 = 7.51$, df = 18, $p > 0.05$), indicating that the effects of the engagement in the motivational environment on the level of self-regulation were not statistically different across the study participants. The proportion reduced in variance at Level-1 compared to the null model was calculated ($R^2_{PRE} = 0.093$), indicating that 9.3% of variance was reduced by adding the Level-1 predictor variable to the null model. The calculated ICC in this model was 0.34.

Finally, the interaction effect between variables in Level-1 and Level-2 was examined (Table 7). As a result of the fixed effects analysis, there was no significant interaction effect between the engagement in two motivational environments and

Table 4. Comparisons between models including each of the personal variables.

Fixed effect	Model 1 Gender			Model 2 Months living in USA			Model 3 EXCELS Experience			Model 4 GenderByEXP		
	Coefficient	SE	t	Coefficient	SE	t	Coefficient	SE	t	Coefficient	SE	t
Intercept (β_{00})	27.44	1.19	22.98**	21.68	6.16	3.52**	19.41	3.12	6.22**	27.45	1.20	22.83**
Gender slope (β_{0i})	−1.27	1.19	−1.06									
MLUS slope (β_{0i})				0.11	0.05	2.14*						
EXP slope (β_{0i})							6.49	2.34	2.78*			
GenderByEXP (β_{0i})										−0.87	.90	−0.97

Random effect	SD	σ^2	χ^2	SD	σ^2	χ^2	SD	σ^2	χ^2	SD	σ^2	χ^2
Level 2 (r_{0i})	4.38	19.14	66.19**	4.48	20.04	72.17**	3.57	12.76	50.34**	4.41	19.47	67.35**
Level 1 (e_{ti})	6.68	44.57		6.66	44.38		6.66	44.31		6.68	44.55	
ICC	0.30			0.31			0.22			0.30		
R^2_{PRE}	03			—			0.35			0.01		

*$p < 0.05$; **$p < 0.001$.

Table 5. Results of the main effects in Level 2 using a mean-as-outcome model.

Fixed effect		Coefficient	SE	t
Intercept (β_{00})		19.06	3.15	6.05**
Gender slope (β_{01})		−3.06	3.15	−0.97
Exp slope (β_{02})		6.66	2.37	2.81*
GenderByEXP slope (β_{03})		1.49	2.37	0.63

Random effect	SD	σ^2	df	χ^2
Participants mean (r_{0i})	3.54	12.54	15	43.09**
Level 1 effect (e_{ti})	6.67	44.49		
ICC (ρ) = 0.22				
R^2_{PRE} = .37				

*$p < 0.05$; **$p < 0.001$.

Table 6. Results of the main effects in Level 1 using a random-coefficient model.

Fixed effect		Coefficient	SE	t
Intercept (β_{00})		27.63	1.19	23.19*
MoEn slope (β_{01})		−3.84	1.17	−3.30**

Random effect	SD	σ^2	df	χ^2
Participants mean (r_{0i})	4.51	20.30	18	81.49*
MoEn slope (r_{1i})	0.92	0.85	18	7.51
Level 1 effect (e_{ti})	6.35	40.31		
ICC (ρ) = 0.34				
R^2_{PRE} = 0.093				

*$p < 0.001$; **$p < 0.01$.

Table 7. Results of the interaction effects between variables in two levels.

Fixed effect		Coefficient	SE	t
Participant means (π_{0i})				
Intercept (β_{00})		18.99	3.14	6.04***
Gender (β_{01})		−2.97	3.14	−0.94
EXP (β_{02})		6.71	2.37	2.83*
GenderByEXP(β_{03})		1.45	2.37	0.61
MoEn slope (π_{1i})				
Intercept (β_{10})		−0.92	3.55	−0.26
Gender (β_{11})		2.29	3.55	0.64
EXP (β_{12})		−2.11	2.69	−0.79
GenderByEXP (β_{13})		−0.31	2.69	−0.12

Random effect	SD	σ^2	df	χ^2
Participants mean (r_{0i})	3.62	13.09	15	47.58***
MoEn slope (r_{1i})	0.33	0.11	15	4.03
Level 1 effect (e_{ti})	6.36	40.45		
ICC (ρ) = 0.49				
R^2_{PRE} (intercept) = 0.35				
R^2_{PRE} (slope) = 0.87				

*$p < 0.05$; ***$p < 0.001$.

participants' variables on increasing self-regulation. The mean of the veteran participants in self-regulation was significantly higher than that of the novice participants while the other Level-2 variables (gender and GenderByEXP) were not significantly associated with the level of self-regulation. The random effects analysis showed that significant variation in the mean self-regulation score of the study participants remained after controlling for gender, EXP and GenderByEXP ($\hat{\tau}_{00}$ = 13.09, $\chi^2 = 47.58$, df = 15, $p < 0.001$). The proportion of variance reduction in both intercept and slope was calculated. Results indicated that 35% of additional variance in the intercept (mean of the study participants' self-regulation) and 87% of additional variance in the slope (regression weight for the self-regulation) were, respectively, explained by adding three Level-2 variables to the random-coefficient model. Finally, the estimated ICC in this model was 0.34.

Discussion

This study examined the effects of participants' personal variables (Level-2) as well as staged motivational environments (Level-1) on autonomous self-regulation among refugee youth. Results revealed that two variables in Level-2 (months resident in the USA and previous experiences in the AAU EXCELS Academy) were significantly associated with the level of autonomous self-regulation. In other words, refugee youth residing longer in the USA appeared to exhibit higher autonomous self-regulation. This result is consistent with the argument of previous studies indicating that opportunities for autonomy in refugee youth may be restricted by long-standing cultural beliefs and collectivism where group goals are more valued over individual's goals (Chakrabarty 2009; Ratner and Hui 2003), and that greater experience and contact with individualistic cultures may increase autonomy. In addition, previous experience in the AAU EXCELS Academy was the strongest predictor of self-regulation among study participants. This result may have been influenced by increased self-esteem and perceived competence of the veteran participants who participated in a pilot study (Kim et al. 2008). Although the gender variable was not a significant predictor in multilevel modelling analysis, the result of an independent sample t-test noted that female participants reported significantly lower levels of autonomous self-regulation than male participants ($t = 2.34$, df = 121, $p < 0.05$, Cohen's $d = 0.60$). The result was not consistent with those of previous studies (Amorose and Anderson-Butcher 2007; Amorose and Horn 2000). This discrepancy may be due to fewer opportunities for autonomous choices afforded to female refugee youth relative to their male counterparts (Espiritu 1999; Ma and Yeh 2005; Stodolska and Livengood 2006). It appears that having opportunities to develop as an autonomous individual is important, especially among female refugee youth.

The environment type was a significant predictor variable in explaining the level of self-regulation of study participants. The self-regulation data collected while study participants were in an ASE showed a higher level of self-regulation than when in a controlled environment. This result was consistent with previous studies verifying the relationship between engaging in an ASE and demonstrating autonomous self-regulation (Hagger, Chatzisarantis, and Biddle 2002; Ntoumanis 2001; Yost and Ellis 2005). Deci and Ryan (2000) posit that individuals engaged in an ASE demonstrate autonomous motivation rather than controlled motivation. Although their proposition has been confirmed by a number of comparison studies, there are no known studies conducted with refugee youth. This study is a beginning for future research examining the relationships under more rigorous conditions and with larger numbers of study participants. The interaction effect between variables in Level-1 and Level-2 was also examined. Results indicate that there was no significant interaction effect between the engagement in two motivational environments and participants' variables on increasing self-regulation. It appears that the effects of the two motivational environments on self-regulation of study participants are consistent regardless of their gender, previous experience in the AAU EXCELS Academy or months residing in the USA. Study participants in the ASE reported significantly higher autonomous self-regulation than those in the controlled motivational environment.

Conclusions

The results of this study provide practitioners from a variety of disciplines with invaluable information regarding the nurturing, development and engagement of refugee youth. Of particular importance is the potential to enrich the lives of refugee youth through participation in a formal leadership development academy. It appears that a staged experience, embedded in an autonomous-supportive environment, will afford refugee youth opportunities to experience autonomy and roles associated with leadership. Cultivating new generations of leaders in refugee families may ensure their stability, upwards mobility and assimilation into the fabric of society. Failure to create a generation of leaders may relegate them to non-contributing roles in a society which values autonomy, freedom and personal achievement. Creating opportunities for leadership development among refugee youth appears to be one way to break the cycle of dependence, social isolation, marginalization and poverty.

In addition, opportunities for practising autonomy anchored in self-determination theory may allow refugee youth to experience successful accomplishment in various aspects of their lives. The mental and psychological health of refugee youth is critical after resettlement. Of specific concern is the high level of depression, anxiety and PTSD, as well as diminished self-esteem, self-efficacy and learned helplessness, in this population (Allwood, Bell-Dolan, and Husain 2002; Lustig et al. 2004; Loughry and Flouri 2001). Evidence indicates that these mental and psychological problems are strongly associated with lower levels of autonomy (Gillespie, Peltzer, and MaClachlan 2000; Kolts, Robinson, and Tracy 2004; Lustig et al. 2004; Steele, van der Hart, and Nijenhuis 2001). Constructing an environment in which levels of autonomy in refugee youth are elevated appears essential.

Notes on contributors

Dr. Kiboum Kim is a Visiting Researcher in the School of Public Health at Indiana University Bloomington, and a Senior Research Associate at the GreenPlay for Research, Education, and Development (GPRED).

Dr. David M. Compton is a Professor Emeritus in the School of Public Health at Indiana University Bloomington, and a Senior Scholar at The Polis Center, Indiana University-Purdue University Indianapolis (IUPUI).

Dr. Bryan McCormick is a Professor in the School of Public Health at Indiana University Bloomington.

References

Aksamit, D. L., and J. L. Rankin. 1993. "Problem-Solving Teams as a Pre-referral Process." *Special Services in the Schools* 7 (1): 1–25. doi:10.1300/J008v07n01_01.

Allwood, M. A., D. Bell-Dolan, and S. A. Husain. 2002. "Children's Trauma and Adjustment Reactions to Violent and Nonviolent War Experiences." *Journal of the American Academy of Child and Adolescent Psychiatry* 41 (4): 450–457. doi:10.1097/00004583-200204000-00018.

Amabile, T. M., P. Goldfarb, and S. C. Brackfield. 1990. "Social Influences on Creativity: Evaluation, Coaction, and Surveillance." *Creativity Research Journal* 3 (1): 6–21. doi:10.1080/10400419009534330.

Amorose, A. J., and D. Anderson-Butcher. 2007. "Autonomy-Supportive Coaching and Self-Determined Motivation in High School and College Athletes: A Test of Self-Determination Theory." *Psychology of Sport and Exercise* 8 (5): 654–670. doi:10.1016/j.psychsport.2006.11.003.

Amorose, A. J., and T. S. Horn. 2000. "Intrinsic Motivation: Relationships with Collegiate Athletes' Gender, Scholarship Status, and Perceptions of Their Coaches' Behavior." *Journal of Sport Exercise Psychology* 22 (1): 63–84.

Assor, A., H. Kaplan, Y. Kanat-Maymon, and G. Roth. 2005. "Directly Controlling Teacher Behaviors as Predictors of Poor Motivation and Engagement in Girls and Boys: The Role of Anger and Anxiety." *Learning and Instruction* 15 (5): 397–413. doi:10.1016/j.learninstruc.2005.07.008.

Assor, A., H. Kaplan, and G. Roth. 2002. "Choice is Good, but Relevance Is Excellent: Autonomy-Enhancing and Suppressing Teacher Behaviors in Predicting Students' Engagement in School Work." *British Journal of Educational Psychology* 72 (2): 261–278. doi:10.1348/000709902158883.

Au, R., D. Watkins, J. Hattie, and P. Alexander. 2009. "Reformulating the Depression Model of Learned Helplessness for Academic Outcomes." *Educational Research Review* 4 (2): 103–117. doi:10.1016/j.edurev.2009.04.001.

Berenson, G., S. Bonura, S. Hunter, L. Webber, L. Myers, and C. Johnson. 1997. "Learned Helplessness with Excess Weight and Other Cardiovascular Risk Factors in Children." *American Journal of Health Behavior* 21: 51–59.

Birman, D., and E. J. Trickett. 2001. "The Process of Acculturation in First Generation Immigrants: A Study of Soviet Jewish Refugee Adolescents and Parents." *Journal of Cross-Cultural Psychology* 32 (4): 456–477. doi:10.1177/0022022101032004006.

Black, A. E., and E. L. Deci. 2000. "The Effects of Student Self-Regulation and Instructor Autonomy Support on Learning in a College-level Natural Science Course: A Self-Determination Theory Perspective." *Science Education* 84 (6): 740–756. doi:10.1002/1098-237X(200011)84:6<740::AID-SCE4>3.0.CO;2-3.

Bloomberg, L., A. Ganey, V. Alba, G. Quintero, and L. A. Alcantara. 2003. "Chicano-Latino Youth Leadership Institute: An Asset-based Program for Youth." *American Journal of Health Behavior* 27: S45–S54. doi:10.5993/AJHB.27.1.s1.5.

Buki, L. P., T. C. Ma, R. D. Strom, and S. K. Strom. 2003. "Chinese Immigrant Mothers of Adolescents: Self-Perceptions of Acculturation Effects on Parenting." *Cultural Diversity & Ethnic Minority Psychology* 9 (2): 127–140. doi:10.1037/1099-9809.9.2.127.

Chakrabarty, S. 2009. "The Influence of National Culture and Institutional Voids on Family Ownership of Large Firms: A Country Level Empirical Study." *Journal of International Management* 15 (1): 32–45. http://ssrn.com/abstract=1151025.

Connell, J. P., and J. G. Wellborn. 1991. "Competence, Autonomy and Relatedness: A Motivational Analysis of Self-System Processes." In *The Minnesota Symposium on Child Psychology*, edited by M. R. Gunnar and L. A. Sroufe, 43–77. Hillsdale, NJ: Erlbaum.

d'Ailly, H. 2003. "Children's Autonomy and Perceived Control in Learning: A Model of Motivation and Achievement in Taiwan." *Journal of Educational Psychology* 95 (1): 84–96. doi:10.1037/0022-0663.95.1.84.

Deci, E. L., and R. M. Ryan. 1985. *Intrinsic Motivation and Self-Determination in Human Behavior*. New York: Plenum.

Deci, E. L., and R. M. Ryan. 2000. "The 'What' and 'Why' of Goal Pursuits: Human Needs and the Self-Determination of Behavior." *Psychological Inquiry* 11 (4): 227–268. doi:10.1207/S15327965PLI1104_01.

Deci, E. L., A. J. Schwartz, L. Sheinman, and R. M. Ryan. 1981. "An Instrument to Assess Adults' Orientations toward Control Versus Autonomy with Children: Reflections on Intrinsic Motivation and Perceived Competence." *Journal of Educational Psychology* 73 (5): 642–650. doi:10.1037/0022-0663.73.5.642.

Derluyn, I., and E. Broekaert. 2007. "Different Perspectives on Emotional and Behavioural Problems in Unaccompanied Refugee Minors." *Ethnicity & Health* 12 (2): 141–162. doi:10.1080/13557850601002296.

Dimmock, C., and A. Walker. 2000. *Future School Administration: Global or Culture Bound?* Hong Kong: The Chinese University Press.

Eccles, J., and J. A. Gootman. 2002. *Community Programs to Promote Youth Development.* Washington, DC: National Academy Press.

Ellis, G., C. Morris, and E. Trunnell. 1995. "Engineering Experiences: The COMPLEX Model of Recreation Leadership." *World Leisure and Recreation* 37 (4): 37–43. doi:10.1080/10261133.1995.9673988.

Erath, S., K. Flanagan, and K. Bierman. 2007. "Social Anxiety and Peer Relations in Early Adolescence: Behavioral and Cognitive Factors." *Journal of Abnormal Child Psychology* 35 (3): 405–416. doi:10.1007/s10802-007-9099-2.

Espiritu, Y. L. 1999. "Gender and Labor in Asian Immigrant Families." *American Behavioral Scientist* 42: 628–647. doi:10.1177/00027649921954390.

Foster, M. 2000. "Positive and Negative Responses to Personal Discrimination: Does Coping Make a Difference?" *The Journal of Social Psychology* 140: 93–106. doi:10.1080/00224540009600448.

Fuligni, A. J., and C. Hardway. 2004. "Preparing Diverse Adolescents for the Transfer to Adulthood." *The Future of Children* 14 (2): 99–116. doi:10.2307/1602796.

Gale, L. A. 2011. *A Bridge between Two Worlds: Leadership among Resettled Sudanese Youth in an American City.* Switzerland: UNHCR. http://www.unhcr.org/4e0dbe039.pdf.

Gillespie, A., K. Peltzer, and M. MaClachlan. 2000. "Returning Refugees: Psychological Problems and Mediators of Mental Health among Malawian Returnees." *Journal of Mental Health* 9 (2): 165–178. doi:10.1080/09638230050009168.

Gordon, R., and M. Gordon. 2008. *Learned Helplessness and School Failure.* Beaumont, CA: Robert & Myrna Gordon. http://www.turned-offchild.com/articles/LearnedHelplessnessandSchoolFailure-Part1.pdf.

Hagger, M. S., N. L. Chatzisarantis, and S. J. Biddle. 2002. "The Influence of Autonomous and Controlling Motives on Physical Activity Intentions within the Theory of Planned Behavior." *British Journal of Health Psychology* 7 (3): 283–297. doi:10.1348/135910702760213689.

Halpern, R. 2002. "A Different Kind of Child Development Institution: The History of After-School Programs for Low-Income Children." *Teachers College Record* 104 (2): 178–211. doi:10.1111/1467-9620.00160.

Harrell-Bond, B. E. 2000. *Are Refugee Camps Good for Children?* Geneva: UNHCR. http://www.unhcr.org/3ae6a0c64.html.

Henley, J., and J. Robinson. 2011. "Mental Health Issues among Refugee Children and Adolescents." *Clinical Psychologist* 15 (2): 51–62. doi:10.1111/j.1742-9552.2011.00024.x.

Hesselbein, F., M. Goldsmith, and R. Beckhard. 1996. *Leader of the Future: New Visions, Strategies, and Practices for the Next Era.* 2nd ed. San Francisco, CA: Jossey-Bass.

Hjern, A., B. Angel, and B. Hoejer. 1991. "Persecution and Behavior: A Report of Refugee Children from Chile." *Child Abuse and Neglect* 15 (3): 239–248. doi:10.1016/0145-2134(91)90068-O.

Jarrett, R., P. Sullivan, and N. Watkins. 2005. "Developing Social Capital through Participation in Organized Youth Programs: Qualitative Insights from Three Programs." *Journal of Community Psychology* 33: 41–56. doi:10.1002/jcop.20038.

Joussemet, M., R. Koestner, N. Lekes, and N. Houlfort. 2004. "Introducing Uninteresting Tasks to Children: A Comparison of the Effects of Rewards and Autonomy Support." *Journal of Personality* 72 (1): 139–166. doi:10.1111/j.0022-3506.2004.00259.x.

Khanlou, N., M. Beiser, E. Cole, M. Freire, I. Hyman, and K. Kilbride. 2002. *Mental Health Promotion among Newcomer Female Youth: Post-Migration Experiences and Self-Esteem.* Ontario, Canada: Status of Women Canada. http://www.swccfc.gc.ca/pubs/pubspr/0662320840/200206_0662320840_e.pdf.

Kim, K., D. M. Compton, and S. Cheng. 2008. *The Effect of the AAU EXCELS Academy Anchored in Self-determination Theory on Self-efficacy, Perceived Competence, and Leadership Skills among Refugee Youth (Ages 14–16).* Salt Lake City: University of Utah.

Kirk, J., and E. Cassity. 2007. "Minimum Standards for Quality Education for Refugee Youth." *Youth Studies Australia* 26 (1): 50–56. http://www.acys.info/journal/issues/v26-n1-2007/summaries/article6.

Knafo, A., and A. Assor. 2007. "Motivation for Agreement with Parental Values: Desirable When Autonomous, Problematic When Controlled." *Motivation Emotion* 31 (3): 232–245. doi:10.1007/s11031-007-9067-8.

Kolts, R. L., A. M. Robinson, and J. J. Tracy. 2004. "The Relationship of Sociotropy and Autonomy to Posttraumatic Cognitions and PTSD Symptomatology in Trauma Survivors." *Journal of Clinical Psychology* 60 (1): 53–63. doi:10.1002/jclp.10193.

Kwak, K. 2003. "Adolescents and Their Parents: A Review of Intergenerational Family Relations for Immigrant and Non-Immigrant Families." *Human Development* 46 (2–3): 15–136. doi:10.1159/000068581.

Lakes, R. 1996. *Youth Development and Critical Education: The Promise of Democratic Action.* New York, NY: SUNY Press.

Lewis, A., E. Huebner, P. Malone, and R. Valois. 2011. "Life Satisfaction and Student Engagement in Adolescents." *Journal of Youth and Adolescence* 40 (3): 249–262. doi:10.1007/s10964-010-9517-6.

Lieber, E., D. Chin, K. Nihira, and I. T. Mink. 2001. "Holding On and Letting Go: Identity and Acculturation Among Chinese Immigrants." *Cultural Diversity and Ethnic Minority Psychology* 7 (3): 247–261. doi:10.1037/1099-9809.7.3.247.

Liebkind, K., I. Jasinskaja-Lahti, and E. Solheim. 2004. "Cultural Identity, Perceived Discrimination, and Parental Support as Determinants of Immigrants' School Adjustments." *Journal of Adolescence Research* 19 (6): 635–656. doi:10.1177/0743558404269279.

Long, T., G. Ellis, E. Trunnell, K. Tatsugawa, and P. Freeman. 2001. "Animating Recreation Experiences Through Face-to-Face Leadership: Efficacy of Two Models." *Journal of Park and Recreation Administration*, 19 (1): 1–22. http://js.sagamorepub.com/jpra/article/view/1582.

Loughry, M., and E. Flouri. 2001. "The Behavioral and Emotional Problems of Former Unaccompanied Refugee Children 3–4 Years after Their Return to Vietnam." *Child Abuse & Neglect* 25 (2): 249–263. doi:10.1016/S0145-2134(00)00240-4.

Lustig, S. L., S. M. Weine, G. N. Saxe, and W. R. Beardslee. 2004. "Testimonial Psychotherapy for Adolescent Refugees: A Case Series." *Transcultural Psychiatry* 41 (1): 31–45. doi:10.1177/1363461504041352.

Ma, P. W., and C. J. Yeh. 2005. "Factors Influencing the Career Decision Status of Chinese American Youth." *Career Development Quarterly* 53 (4): 337–347. doi:10.1002/j.2161-0045.2005.tb00664.x.

Mackenzie, C., C. McDowell, and E. Pittaway. 2007. "Beyond 'Do No Harm': The Challenge of Constructing Ethical Relationships in Refugee Research." *Journal of Refugee Studies* 20 (2): 299–319. doi:10.1093/jrs/fem008.

Marshall, E. K., and G. D. Ellis. 2003. "Animating Recreation Experiences: Effects of Behavior-Specific Verbal Feedback on Experiences of First-Time Skiers." *Journal of Park and Recreation Administration* 21 (3): 120–139. http://js.sagamorepub.com/jpra/article/view/1502.

Maxwell, S. E., and H. D. Delaney. 2004. *Designing Experiments and Analyzing Data: A Model Comparison Perspective.* 2nd ed. Mahwah, NJ: Lawrence Erlbaum Associates.

McLaughlin, M., M. Irby, and J. Langman. 1994. *Urban Sanctuaries: Neighborhood Organizations in the Lives and Futures of Inner-City Youth.* San Francisco, CA: Jossey-Bass.

Mesch, G. S. 2002. "Between Spatial and Social Segregation among Immigrants." *International Migration Review* 36 (3): 912–934. doi:10.1111/j.1747-7379.2002.tb00109.x.

Mesch, G. S., H. Turjeman, and G. Fishman. 2008. "Perceived Discrimination and the Well-being of Immigrant Adolescents." *Journal of Youth and Adolescents* 37 (5): 592–604. doi:10.1007/s10964-007-9210-6.

Murray, L., J. Cohen, B. Ellis, and A. Mannarino. 2008. "Cognitive Behavioral Therapy for Symptoms of Trauma and Traumatic Grief in Refugee Youth." *Refugee Mental Health* 17 (3): 585–604. doi:10.1016/j.chc.2008.02.003.

National Child Traumatic Stress Network. 2005. *Mental Health Interventions for Refugee Children in Resettlement: Child and Adolescent Refugee Mental Health.* http://www.nctsnet.org/nctsn_assets/pdfs/promising_practices/MH_Interventions_for_Refugee_Children.pdf.

Ntoumanis, N. 2001. "A Self-Determination Approach to the Understanding of Motivation in Physical Education." *British Journal of Educational Psychology* 71 (2): 225–242. doi:10.1348/000709901158497.

Oppedal, B., E. Roysamb, and D. L. Sam. 2004. "The Effect of Acculturation and Social Support on Change in Mental Health among Young Immigrants." *International Journal of Behavioral Development* 28 (6): 481–494. doi:10.1080/01650250444000126.

Papadopoulos, R. K. 2001. "Refugee Families: Issues of Systemic Supervision." *Journal of Family Therapy* 23 (4): 405–422. doi:10.1111/1467-6427.00193.

Pelletier, L. G., M. S. Fortier, R. J. Vallerand, and N. M. Briére. 2001. "Associations among Perceived Autonomy Support, Forms of Self-regulation and Persistence: A Prospective Study." *Motivation and Emotion* 25 (4): 279–306. doi:10.1023/A:1014805132406.

Pelletier, L., and D. Markland. 2004. *Exercise Self-Regulation Questionnaire (SRQ-E).* http://www.psych.rochester.edu/SDT/index.html.

Perkins, D. F., L. M. Borden, F. A. Villarruel, A. Carlton-Hug, M. R. Stone, and J. G. Keith. 2007. "Why Ethnic Minority Urban Youth Choose to Participate-or Not to Participate." *Youth and Society* 38 (4): 420–442. doi:10.1177/0044118X06295051.

Peterson, C., S. F. Maier, and M. S. P. Seligman. 1993. *Learned Helplessness: A Theory for the Age of Personal Control.* New York: Oxford University Press.

Pynoos, R. S., J. D. Kinzie, and M. Gordon. 2001. "Children, Adolescent, and Families Exposed to Torture and Related Trauma." In *The Mental Health Consequences of Torture,* edited by E. Gerrity, T. M. Keane, and T. Tuma, 211–225. New York: Kluwer Academic/Plenum Publications.

Ratner, C., and L. Hui. 2003. "Theoretical and Methodological Problems in Cross-Cultural Psychology." *Journal for the Theory of Social Behavior* 33 (1): 67–94. doi:10.1111/1468-5914.00206.

Raudenbush, S. W., and A. S. Bryk. 2002. *Hierarchical Linear Models: Applications and Data Analysis Methods.* 2nd ed. Thousand Oaks, CA: Sage.

Reeve, J. 2005. *Understanding Motivation and Emotion.* 4th ed. Hoboken, NJ: John Wiley & Sons.

Roark, M. F. 2008. "Relationships among Selected Features of Camps, the Nature of Interactions between and Characteristics of Camp Personnel and Campers, and Campers' Acquisition." PhD diss., College of Health, University of Utah.

Rossman, J. R., and B. E. Schlatter. 2008. *Recreation Programming: Designing Leisure Experiences.* 5th ed. Champaign, IL: Sagamore Publishing.

Ryan, R. M., and J. P. Connell. 1989. "Perceived Locus of Causality and Internalization: Examining Reasons for Acting in Two Domains." *Journal of Personality and Social Psychology* 57: 749–761. http://www.selfdeterminationtheory.org/SDT/documents/1989_RyanConnell.pdf.

Ryan, R. M., and E. L. Deci. 2000. "Self-determination Theory and the Facilitation of Intrinsic Motivation, Social Development, and Well-being." *American Psychologist* 55 (1): 68–78. doi:10.1037/0003-066X.55.1.68.

Ryan, R. M., and E. L. Deci. 2007. "Active Human Nature: Self-Determination Theory and the Promotion and Maintenance of Sport, Exercise, and Health." In *Intrinsic Motivation and Self-Determination in Exercise and Sport,* edited by M. S. Hagge and N. L. D. Chatzisarantis, 1–19. Champaign, IL: Human Kinetics.

Ryan, R. M., and Grolnick, W. S. 1986. "Origins and Pawns in the Classroom: Self-Report and Projective Assessment of Individual Differences in Children's Perceptions." *Journal of Personality and Social Psychology* 50 (3): 550–558. doi:10.1037/0022-3514.50.3.550.

Ryan, R. M., S. Rigby, and K. King. 1993. "Two Types of Religious Internalization and Their Relations to Religious Orientation and Mental Health." *Journal of Personality and Social Psychology* 65 (3): 586–596. doi:10.1037/0022-3514.65.3.586.

Sato, T., and D. McCann. 1997. "Vulnerability Factors in Depression: The Facets of Sociotropy and Autonomy." *Journal of Psychopathology and Behavioral Assessment* 19 (1): 41–62. doi:10.1007/BF02263228.

Sideridis, G. D. (2003). "On the Origin of Helplessness Behaviour of Students with Learning Disabilities: Avoidance Motivation?" *International Journal of Educational Research* 39 (4–5): 497–517. doi:10.1016/j.ijer.2004.06.011.

Sommers, M. 2002. *Crossing Lines: Magnets and Mobility among Southern Sudanese. Basic Education and Policy Support (BEPS) Activity.* Atlanta, GA: United States Agency for International Development. http://www.beps.net/publications/SUDAN-Crossing%20Lines-Magnets%20and%20Mobility.pdf.

Standage, M., J. L. Duda, and N. Ntoumanis. 2005. "A Test of Self-Determination Theory in School Physical Education." *British Journal of Educational Psychology* 75 (3): 411–433. doi:10.1348/000709904X22359.

Steele, K., O. van der Hart, and E. R. S. Nijenhuis. 2001. "Dependency in the Treatment of Complex Posttraumatic Stress Disorder and Dissociative Disorders." *Journal of Trauma and Dissociation* 2 (4): 79–116. doi:10.1300/J229v02n04_05.

Stodolska, M., and J. S. Livengood. 2006. "The Influence of Religion on the Leisure Behavior of American Muslim Immigrants." *Journal of Leisure Research* 38: 293–320. http://search.ebscohost.com/login.aspx?direct=true&db=f5h&AN=21801650&site=ehost-live.

Taylor, J., and R. J. Turner. 2002. "Perceived Discrimination, Social Stress, and Depression in the Transition to Adulthood: Racial Contrasts." *Social Psychology Quarterly* 65 (3): 213–225. doi:10.2307/3090120.

Thomas, M., and E. S. van Mierop. 2004. "Convention Plus? Better Protection for Refugees." *Forced Migration Review* 20: 36. http://www.isn.ethz.ch/Digital-Library/Publications/Detail/?ots591=0c54e3b3-1e9c-be1e-2c24-a6a8c7060233&lng=en&id=129777.

Tiltnes, A. 2005. *Falling Behind. A Brief on the Living Conditions of Palestinian Refugees in Lebanon.* Oslo: FAFO Institute for Applied Social Science.

UNHCR. 2011a. *Global Trends 2010.* Geneva, Switzerland: UNHCR. http://www.unhcr.org/4dfa11499.html.

UNHCR. 2011b. *Challenges Faced by Young Refugees and Asylum Seekers in Accessing Their Social Rights and Their Integration, While in Transition to Adulthood.* Consultative Meeting Report. France: European Youth Centre Strasbourg. http://www.coe.int/t/dg4/youth/Source/Resources/Documents/2011_Report_CM_Young_Refugees_Asylum_Seekers_en.pdf.

United States Citizenship and Immigration Services. 2008. *Immigration and Nationality Act.* http://www.fourmilab.ch/uscode/8usc/www/t8–12-I-1101.html.

United States Department of Homeland Security. 2011. *Annual Flow Report: Refugees and Asylees: 2010.* http://www.dhs.gov/xlibrary/assets/statistics/publications/ois_rfa_fr_2010.pdf.

Vansteenkiste, M., Z. Mingming, L. Willy, and B. Soenens. 2005. "Experiences of Autonomy and Control Among Chinese Learners: Vitalizing or Immobilizing?" *Journal of Educational Psychology* 97 (3): 468–483. doi:10.1037/0022-0663.97.3.468.

Weisskirch, R. S., and S. A. Alva. 2002. "Language Brokering and the Acculturation of Latino Children." *Hispanic Journal of Behavioral Sciences* 24 (3): 369–378.

Wilkinson, L. 2002. "Factors Influencing the Academic Success of Refugee Youth in Canada." *Journal of Youth Studies* 5 (2): 173–193.

World Health Organization. 2005. *Mental and Social Health During and after Acute Emergencies Emerging Consensus?* http://www.searo.who.int/LinkFiles/List_of_Guidelines_for_Health_Emergency_Menta_social-health.pdf.

Yeh, C. J., A. B. Kim, S. T. Pituc, and M. Atkins. 2008. "Poverty, Loss, and Resilience: The Story of Chinese Immigrant Youth." *Journal of Counseling Psychology* 55 (1): 34–48.

Yoshikawa, L. 2005. *Between a Rock and a Hard Place: Burmese Asylum Seekers in Thailand.* Las Vegas, NV: RSDwatch. http://www.rsdwatch.org/index_files/Page1525.htm.

Yost, E., and G. E. Ellis. 2005. "Effect of Self-Determination Theory-Based Recreation Activity-staging on Vitality and Affinity toward Nature among Youth in a Residential

Treatment Program." *Residential Treatment for Children and Youth* 23 (1–2): 5–26. http://www.informaworld.com/openurl?genre=article&id=doi:10.1300/J007v23n01_02.

Zabaneh, J., G. Watt, and C. O'Donnell. 2008. "Living and Health Conditions of Palestinian Refugees in an Unofficial Camp in the Lebanon: A Cross-sectional Survey." *Journal of Epidemiology & Community Health* 62 (2): 91–97.

Zeldin, S., and L. Camino. 1999. "Youth Leadership: Linking Research and Program Theory to Exemplary Practice." *New Designs for Youth Development* 15 (1): 10–15. http://4h.uwex.edu/yig/documents/YouthLeadership-LinkingResearchandProgramTheorytoExemplaryPractice.pdf.

Zhou, M. 2001. "Straddling Different Worlds: The Acculturation of Vietnamese Refugee Children." In *Ethnicities: Children of Immigrants in America*, edited by R. G. Rumbaut and A. Portes, 187–227. Berkeley, CA: University of California Press.

Enhancing communication between a person with TBI and a significant other through arts: pilot project

Hélène Carbonneau[a], Guylaine Le Dorze[b], France Joyal[c] and Marie-Josée Plouffe[c]

[a]Département de Loisir, Culture et Tourisme, Université du Québec à Trois-Rivières, Trois-Rivières, Québec, Canada; [b]École d'Orthophonie et d'Audiologie, Faculté de Médecine, Université de Montréal, Montréal, Québec, Canada; [c]Département de Philosophie et des Arts, Université du Québec à Trois-Rivières, Trois-Rivières, Québec, Canada

The neurological consequences following a traumatic brain injury (TBI) greatly affect the person's daily life as well as that of the supporting relatives who often feel powerless. The social integration of people suffering from TBI is a long-term situation. TBI often involves communication and behavioural disorders that become limitations to social participation. In general, interventions focus on reducing the individual's difficulties and do not consider strengthening their potential. Leisure, notably arts, has been found to assist in adapting to the loss of autonomy and enhancing social reintegration. This paper proposes a new approach focused on strengthening potential through artistic recreational activities as a medium for improving communication between a person with a TBI and his/her relative. A pre-experimental study was conducted with a group of dyads of persons with TBI and their significant other ($n = 5$ dyads). Unexpected quantitative changes were found on the Perception of Relationship and Activities Scale, more specifically on the sharing pleasant events sub-scale which decreased for the significant other group, as well as decreases on the feelings, values and feasibility of this sub-scale. However, the qualitative results revealed interesting impacts of the programme on self-realization and relationships. These data will allow us to further test the programme in an experimental study.

Introduction

In the USA, emergency visits, hospitalizations and deaths due to traumatic brain injury (TBI) are estimated at 1.7 million per year (Centers for Disease Control and Prevention 2013). The annual rate of hospitalizations for TBI is 43 per 100,000 in Quebec (Institut National en Santé Publique du Québec 2012). TBI is the main cause of death among adults under 35 years of age and it also represents a major cause of disability. Although the consequences of TBI vary, they may bring about changes for the family as well as social, academic and professional changes for the person affected (McDonald 2013; Perlesz, Kinsella, and Crowe 2000). Personality changes can impact on social abilities and relationships (Demakis et al. 2007). Role changes and financial consequences can create problems with self (Douglas 2013). The social integration of people with TBI may be a long-term issue for all concerned (Lefebvre, Cloutier, and Levert 2008). Caregivers may find the situation emotionally demanding. Therefore, people with TBI and their significant others should receive support in order to maintain a positive relationship with one another and offset the negative consequences of TBI (Foster et al. 2012; Rietdijk, Togher, and Power 2012).

TBI may involve cognitive-linguistic disorders, difficulties in respecting the unwritten rules of interpersonal communication and, less frequently, other communication disorders such as aphasia or dysarthria. Any of these communication disorders can become a barrier in daily life and in relationships, even for the significant others and caregivers (Ylvisaker, Turkstra, and Coelho 2005). Communication problems, ineffective support, and behavioural issues may all contribute to poor social integration for the person with TBI (Le Dorze and Brassard 1995; Ylvisaker, Turkstra, and Coelho 2005). Caregivers (family members, spouse or friends) also experience changes in their relationship with their relative (Turner et al. 2010). They may become socially withdrawn as a consequence of the role of support to an individual with behavioural and communication disabilities (Lefebvre, Désilets, and Ndakengurukiye 2004).

Rehabilitation

Rehabilitation generally focuses on reducing the disabilities people with TBI may experience (Ylvisaker, Turkstra, and Coelho 2005). Rehabilitation programmes rarely also include families and caregivers as dyads receiving support for improving communication, relationships and social outcomes. Moreover, few approaches are based on the idea of strengthening the potential of communication between the person with TBI and his/her significant other. The project on which this paper is based proposes a new approach focused on strengthening potential by providing a shared leisure experience, based on arts, as a medium for improving communication between the person with TBI and his/her significant other.

Role of leisure

Involvement in leisure activities may help counter the negative consequences of TBI. Research literature is replete with studies indicating the positive impacts of leisure, both for healthy people and for people living with disabilities (Carbonneau et al. 2011; Devine 2004; Driver, Brown, and Peterson 1991; Zumbo 2003). Participation in leisure has a positive influence on stress management (Iwasaki, MacTavish, and MacKay 2005). In parallel with recreation, artistic medium is often used for therapeutic purposes. Even though the goals of engaging in art or physical activities may differ, the benefits identified by the participants who engage in such activities are similar. Many studies reinforce the importance of leisure in rehabilitation, reintegration and social well-being of people with disabilities (Lammel 2003; Rhondali et al. 2007). Hutchinson et al. (2003) demonstrated the role of leisure in the coping process following traumatic injury. LoBello et al. (2003) showed that social integration was linked to greater general life satisfaction for people with TBI. They stated that the quality of life after the injury was more related 'to a healthy psychological functioning rather than the degree of physical impairment' (298). Achieving a healthy and productive lifestyle seemed to be related to overall life satisfaction (Corrigan et al. 2001; Steadman-Pare et al. 2001). The social support and interpersonal consequences of participation in leisure also play an important role in the psychological well-being of people with TBI (Lammel 2003). According to

Lammel (2003), leisure has a positive effect regarding the social relations of the person with TBI.

The positive impacts of leisure for rehabilitation and social reintegration have been found to contribute to the person's well-being (Lammel 2003; Hutchinson et al. 2003). Artistic activities may be a particularly good form of recreation when trying to adapt to an illness or a traumatic injury. Reynolds (2003) found that the artistic pursuits of women living with cancer enabled them to reconnect with their former inner self. Art was therefore a means of growth and it enabled the development of a positive identity through the emergence of symbolic reintegration and new abilities in coping with the loss of something important. Indeed, involvement in art allowed participants to express their 'personal story' and to find a positive way to move forward and achieve their aspirations (Reynolds, Vivat, and Prior 2008). Artistic activities can also help bring back expertise, social status and self-esteem through tangible productions and help gain skills and knowledge acquired through lectures and classes. In their book, *Art until the end of life,* Rhondali et al. (2007) explained that artistic recreational activities facilitated the expression of emotions and psychological concerns. Art therapy has been found to significantly contribute to coping, reintegration and management of important changes brought about by a significant loss of autonomy (David 1999).

The programme proposed in the study on which this paper is based aims to improve communication within dyads comprised of an individual with TBI and a significant other by exposing them together to artistic activities (drawing, theatre and dance). These activities could be conducive to reviving the relationship between the members of the dyad, a relationship that may have been altered because of role changes associated with caregiving and loss of independence, as well as changes in communication. It was hypothesized that improved communication during these experiences in art (drawing, theatre and dance) could have beneficial effects on both the caregiver and the person with TBI according to the cognitive potential of the artistic activity (Goodman 1968, 1992) coupled with the cognitive partnership (Barth 2002). We did not use a traditional TBI rehabilitation technique nor did we emphasize artistic training of any sort. Instead, the project aimed at bringing participants together to share the present moment in a pleasant and creative context. It allowed both members of the dyad to participate in the process of co-construction of meaning within each activity. When recognizing themselves and their partner during the new activities they were involved with, they were able to take advantage of the present moment (Stern 2004), and thus have a better appreciation of their relationship. To our knowledge, no similar project was previously undertaken.

Objectives

The objectives of the study were to:

(1) Develop an arts programme that was adapted to dyads of people with TBI and a significant other which would provide a supportive approach to communication.
(2) Evaluate the impacts of this arts programme (drawing, theatre and dance) on the person with TBI and a significant other.

Methods

Participants

The study participants were persons with TBI and a significant other (family members or friends). By definition, significant others offered regular support in the form of at least one weekly visit. All were community living individuals. Inclusion criteria for participants with TBI were as follows: reported moderate-to-severe TBI, no other neurological or psychiatric hospitalization required within the past year and no current depression. Participants were recruited from people attending a TBI association and the community organization where the programme was held. A convenience sample of six dyads accepted to participate. One dyad dropped out after two weeks because the person with TBI was too tired to attend the programme in the evening.

Study design

A pre-experimental study with mixed methods was conducted with a group of five dyads of persons with TBI and their identified significant other. The programme was offered in a community organization in a city of about 100,000 residents. The Ethics Committee of Research of the Université du Québec à Trois-Rivières approved the project. The project was undertaken from September to December 2009.

Participants committed to an eight-week programme during which they participated in different artistic activities such as drawing, theatre and dance for two hours each week. The development of this programme was based on the idea that the arts programme should have a positive impact on the general well-being of a person with TBI and his/her caregiver. The impact of the intervention was hypothesized to change the quality of communication and improve the perception of their relationship on a daily basis. Figure 1 illustrates this framework.

Programme description

The arts (drawing, theatre and dance) programme aimed to provide participants with shared pleasant experiences through artistic activities within a group environment where the roles of caregiver and care receiver were not emphasized. In fact, the participants were all expected to contribute fully as related individuals or as friends.

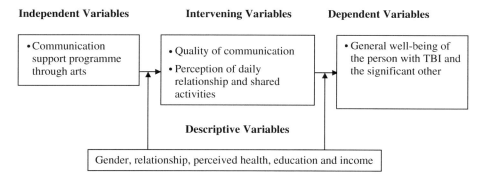

Figure 1. Illustration of variables framework.

The art specialists and the facilitator were trained in appropriate facilitative communication by a speech-language therapist. The training focused on Kagan et al.'s (2001) principles, namely that a communication disorder hides the person's competence and that appropriate communication attitudes will enable an individual to reveal his/her competence. Two of the art specialists were professors in the arts field and involved as researchers in the project. One is a professor in the field of drama and the other one specialized in dance. The third art specialist was an experienced art therapist with a master's degree.

The programme content was based on an approach focused on the process of participation and the experience, rather than on outcomes themselves or the product of the art session. The goal of the first two-hour session was for the participants to get to know one another. Then, various art mediums were explored over the next six weeks in two consecutive sessions each: drawing, theatre and dance. Each session involved activities or exercises that focused on different means of communication using the medium. At the end of each session, a research assistant encouraged the participants to reflect and discuss the session in the absence of the arts specialist of the day. The last session wrapped up the programme.

Data collection

The following procedures were used for data collection. For the quantitative data, all of the participants answered several standardized measures described below. For the qualitative data, open-ended interviews were conducted with each participant after the completion of the programme.

Quantitative part

For the quantitative part, an initial evaluation of participants was completed two weeks before the beginning of the programme by a trained research assistant. The participants' consent was obtained at that moment. Participants were re-evaluated at the end of the programme by the same research assistant.

Dependent variables

Well-being. The French version of the *General Well Being Schedule* (Dupuy 1978) was used to assess well-being. This questionnaire contained 18 items measuring six dimensions: anxiety, depression, positive well-being, control of emotions, vitality and general health. The first 14 responses were evaluated with a Likert scale of 6 points (0–5), and the last four responses were measured using a 10-point scale, which yielded a score ranging from 0 to 110. A higher score was associated with better well-being. This scale was validated with a French-speaking population and had very good psychometric properties (Bravo, Gaulin, and Dubois 1996). The intra-class correlation coefficient related to the test–retest reliability was 0.82 with a confidence interval 95% ranging from 0.71 to 0.89. Internal consistency rose to 0.92. The average correlation of an item with the total score reached 0.66. The inter-item correlations were all positive and varied from 0.22 to 0.69 (Bravo, Gaulin, and Dubois 1996).

Intervening variables

Communication. The Relational Communication Scale (RCS) (Burgoon and Hale 1987; Hale, Burgoon, and Householder 2005) measured relational messages present during a conversation defining an interpersonal relationship. A translated version in Quebec-French, showing good reliability, was used (Salois-Bellerose, Croteau, and Le Dorze 2008). Participants indicated agreement with 40 statements associated with various dimensions of relational communication: intimacy, dominance and composure. Cronbach's alpha was between 0.88 and 0.93.

Participants were asked to rate the previous week's conversations with their partner, both pre- and post-project on a single sheet of paper. Participants were allowed to respond to the post-test while seeing their first responses in the pre-test. This approach was used successfully by the creators of the Communication Effectiveness Index (CETI) in that seeing one's previous responses reduces variability and errors associated with poor recall (Lomas et al. 1989). Participants rated themselves and their partner separately.

The LaTrobe Communication Questionnaire (LTCQ) (Douglas, O'Flaherty, and Snow 2000) was designed to determine the frequency of communication problems as perceived by individuals with TBI and by their relatives. This tool had satisfactory psychometric properties (Cronbach's alpha = 0.8596) (Douglas, O'Flaherty, and Snow 2000). The researchers developed and used a Quebec-French translation using the reverse translation procedure. An example of a stimulus question was: 'Use a lot of vague or empty words such as "you know what I mean" instead of the right word?'

The LTCQ was administered pre- and post-intervention, and the scores recorded by each participant during the first administration were provided for the second completion, again to minimize the error rate. Participants evaluated themselves and their partner, as speakers, separately during this research project.

Perception of daily shared activities. An attitude scale based on the Osgood method (Leclerc, Montminy, and Noiseux 1989) was used to document how the participants perceived their relationship in terms of maintaining the relationship, doing activities together and shared pleasant events. Three attitude-related components (maintaining the relationship, doing activities together and shared pleasant event) were measured for value (useless, significant), feasibility (easy, difficult) and perception (pleasant, unpleasant) associated with each of these sub-scales. The 'value' dimension illustrated the importance the person attributed to the component. The 'feasibility' dimension described how much the person considered it possible to realize the component. The 'perception' dimension considered pleasantness of the action related to the component of the scale. Each dimension was measured with at least three pairs of adjectives using a 7-level scale.

Descriptive variables

The perceived health of caregivers was evaluated using a single item from the Quebec Health and Social Survey of 1998. The question read as follows: 'Compared to other people your age, would you say your health is: excellent, good, fair or poor?' A socio-demographic questionnaire comprised of items such as education level and income was administered at the pre-test stage.

Quantitative data collection and analysis

A trained research assistant who was not involved in the arts programme aided the participants in responding to the various questionnaires as required. Data collection was held either at their homes or at the university depending on participants' preference. The research assistant was trained with the different measurement tools by two of the research team members.

Participants were characterized using descriptive statistics on all the measures. The effects of the intervention were evaluated by comparing the pre- and post-test data on all the measures using the Wilcoxon signed ranks test (Siegel and Castellan 1988), considering the small number of participants.

Qualitative part. Each participant was interviewed separately at their home or at the university depending on the participant's choice, in order to understand the impacts of their participation in the programme both on themselves and on the dyad. An interview guide was developed for the purpose of this study based upon the insights gained from reviewing the literature. Open-ended questions were formulated on how the programme activities had affected the participants and their dyad. These interviews were conducted, recorded and transcribed by a trained research assistant.

All transcripts were analysed using a content analysis based on Paillé and Mucchielli (2012). This method consisted of systematically locating, grouping and examining the components being addressed. Rigorous data analysis was performed through cross validation by three different researchers (one in the arts field, one in speech therapy and one from the leisure domain). Each of the researchers identified the major themes and sub-themes separately. Following this step, the research team discussed and compared the researchers' analyses until consensus was reached.

Participants

Of the 12 subjects recruited, at the start of the study, 10 completed the entire research programme and attended all sessions. Participants with TBI were all men. There were three women and two men among the significant others. The age range was between 21 and 40 years for the participants with TBI and 14–65 years for the significant others. There were three father and child dyads, one dyad of spouses and one of friends. Table 1 summarizes the participants' socio-demographic characteristics.

Results

Quantitative analyses

The goal of the programme, which was to enhance the general well-being of the participants, was not demonstrated. Although the scores of both groups appeared to change in opposite directions, none of the comparisons reached statistical significance. The large standard deviations reflect high levels of variability within each group. Variability combined with a small sample size did not allow the detection of differences on most measures. Table 2 presents these results.

On the Perception of Relationship and Activities Scale, total scores did not differ on the post-test as compared to the pre-test. However, some statistical differences emerged on the shared pleasant activities scales. Significant others had lower scores on this sub-scale after completing the programme as compared to before. Results are

Table 1. Participants' characteristics.

Variables	Persons with TBI	Significant others
Gender		
Women	0	3
Men	5	2
Relation		
Spouse	1	1
Child	2	1
Father	1	2
Friend	1	1
Age		
< 20	0	1
21–30	2	1
31–40	3	1
41 and over	0	2
Education level		
Elementary	1	0
High school	3	2
College	1	2
University	0	1
Income (CAD $)		
< 10,000	0	2
11,000–29,999	2	1
30,000–49,999	3	1
50,000–69,999	0	0
> 70,000	0	1
Perceived health		
Excellent	0	1
Good	2	2
Average	1	2
Poor	2	0

displayed in Table 3. This was unexpected and revealed that significant others had a less positive perception of sharing pleasant events with the person with TBI after the programme.

The results from the dimensions of the sub-scale scores shown in Table 4 indicated some statistically significant differences. With respect to the sharing pleasant events sub-scale, persons with TBI had lower scores on associated values, significant others also scored lower on the feasibility measure and associated feelings were lower again for this group. These results were also unexpected. All other comparisons did not attain statistical significance.

Although visual inspection of results may suggest a tendency for the means of the significant other of people with TBI to fluctuate in opposite directions following their participation in the programme, the small number of subjects did not allow us

Table 2. Results for general well-being.

Variables	Pre-test	Post-test	p
General well-being (/110)			
Persons with TBI	67.8 ± 16.2	77.2 ± 8.70	0.22
Significant others	71.6 ± 7.73	65.8 ± 13.7	0.35

Table 3. Results of perception of relationship, activities, and pleasant events total scores and sub-scales scores.

Variables	$N = 5$ per group	Pre-test	Post-test	p
Perception of relationship, activities and pleasant events score total (/27)	Persons with TBI	16.0±1.4	15.8±2.4	0.89
	Significant others	17.6±0.7	16.5±2.2	0.35
Sub-scale scores				
Maintaining the daily relationship sub-total (/9)	Persons with TBI	5.1±0.8	5.1±0.8	1
	Significant others	5.6±0.8	5.5±0.9	0.89
Doing shared activities sub-total (/9)	Persons with TBI	5.1±0.6	5.4±1.0	0.79
	Significant others	5.7±0.3	5.4±0.7	0.47
Sharing pleasant events sub-total (/9)	Persons with TBI	5.8±0.1	5.4±0.7	0.23
	Significant others	6.3±0.4	5.5±0.8*	0.04

*$p < 0.05$ (Wilcoxon test).

to use an ANOVA to test group and time differences together, which would have been the best strategy for detecting potential interactions.

None of the pre- versus post-test comparisons on the LTCQ had significance. Scores remained about the same over time. Although not specifically tested, we can

Table 4. Results from the dimensions of sub-scale scores regarding perception of relationship, activities and pleasant events scale.

Variables		Pre-test	Post-test	p
Maintaining the daily relationship				
Associated values	Persons with TBI	5.3±1.2	5.4±1.0	1
	Significant others	6.2±1.1	5.8±1.2	0.41
Feasibility	Persons with TBI	5.0±0.8	5.2±1.1	1
	Significant others	6.0±0.9	5.3±1.0	0.22
Associated feelings	Persons with TBI	5.0±1.3	4.9±1.0	0.69
	Significant others	5.0±1.2	5.5±1.0	0.47
Doing shared activities				
Associated values	Persons with TBI	5.6±1.5	5.5±1.5	0.69
	Significant others	6.3±0.5	5.8±1.0	0.11
Feasibility	Persons with TBI	4.9±0.9	5.1±1.2	0.66
	Significant others	5.0±0.3	5.2±0.8	0.58
Associated feelings	Persons with TBI	4.9±1.0	5.5±1.0	0.46
	Significant others	5.8±0.5	5.4±0.6	0.10
Sharing pleasant events				
Associated values	Persons with TBI	6.2±0.8	5.3±0.6*	0.04
	Significant others	6.5±0.4	6.2±0.8	0.41
Feasibility	Persons with TBI	5.7±0.6	5.3±1.3	0.69
	Significant others	6.0±0.8	5.2±1.0*	0.04
Associated feelings	Persons with TBI	5.6±0.3	5.5±0.6	0.5
	Significant others	6.4±0.5	5.4±0.8*	0.04

*$p < 0.05$ (Wilcoxon test).

note that the scores pertaining to the participants with TBI were 5–10 points higher on average than those of participants without TBI, indicating that this instrument was sensitive to the general differences in communicative behaviours associated with brain injury (Tables 5 and 6).

None of the pre- versus post-test comparisons were statistically significant on the three sub-scales of Intimacy, Dominance or Composure of the Relational Communication Scale (Salois-Bellerose, Croteau, and Le Dorze 2008).

Table 5. Results of the LaTrobe communication questionnaire.

	Pre-test	Post-test	p
Participants with TBI			
Self-evaluated	61.6 ± 2.8	65.8 ± 5.9	0.14
Evaluated by partner	64.8 ± 18.1	62.0 ± 9.9	0.34
Significant others			
Self-evaluated	53.2 ± 9.4	52.2 ± 0.9	0.59
Evaluated by partner with TBI	55.6 ± 7.0	53.2 ± 7.2	0.47

Table 6. Results of the three relational communication sub-scales.

	Pre-test	Post-test	p
Intimacy sub-scale			
Participants with TBI			
Self-evaluated	5.8 ± 0.8	5.5 ± 0.8	0.29
Evaluated by partner	5.6 ± 0.7	5.4 ± 0.6	0.18
Significant others			
Self-evaluated	5.5 ± 0.7	5.6 ± 0.8	0.29
Evaluated by partner with TBI	5.5 ± 1.2	5.6 ± 0.9	0.72
Dominance sub-scale			
Participants with TBI			
Self-evaluated	4.1 ± 1.3	4.5 ± 0.9	0.14
Evaluated by partner	4.3 ± 1.0	4.3 ± 0.7	0.59
Significant others			
Self-evaluated	5.4 ± 0.8	5.4 ± 0.7	0.66
Evaluated by partner with TBI	5.0 ± 0.2	4.9 ± 0.7	0.72
Composure sub-scale			
Participants with TBI			
Self-evaluated	5.8 ± 1.6	5.4 ± 1.2	0.14
Evaluated by partner	5.1 ± 1.1	5.3 ± 1.0	1
Significant others			
Self-evaluated	3.9 ± 1.0	5.0 ± 1.0	0.47
Evaluated by partner with TBI	5.1 ± 1.3	5.1 ± 0.7	0.32

Qualitative analyses

The qualitative analyses revealed that participants underwent a transformation around their personal identities, their perception of their partner and a renewal of their relationship. This qualitative data provided clearer answers to the question of the impacts of the programme than the standardized questionnaires. These finding are exposed below. Please note that quotes were translated from French by the authors.

Participants developed a sense of self-realization through arts activities. This sense was strongly expressed by everyone. One participant explained: 'I would have liked to do more [. . .] but globally, I am proud of my performance' (TBI 4).

The various levels of experience associated with the participation in the programme provided participants with a new consciousness about their relationship and allowed some of them to redefine their relationship. Not only did participants get out of their house, they spent more time together, they had fun together, and were able to 'see' their partner, as well as themselves, differently. Moreover, the fact that all participants were doing something new in a new environment, allowed both members of the dyad to re-discover one another: 'The possibility to get to know each other in a new way and to see the other through a different lens that we did not use daily' (TBI 3). Some were proud of having improved their relationship: 'It is not new activities that were incorporated in our life, but it is the relationship that changed. Relationships were easier' (TBI 3).

This re-acquaintance was not always expressed as a pleasant experience but as a discovery of new feelings. 'It even gave me lots and lots of new feelings. That brought me to feel new things in a day, and in a new way' (TBI 4). This participant also felt different with respect to his father. 'I feel more present in his active life [talking about his father]'.

Another participant spoke of how, through the activities, his self was revealed to his partner and how the partner's identity also became clearer:

> Here I saw my partner in another context of activities, [...] you see the other [person] displaying other abilities and me too, I am ... performing in this too. You communicate and you see other common interests in that and through that. (TBI 3)

Moreover, this mutual revealing of self may have provided the opportunity for a greater self-awareness of their potential and allowed them to project themselves in future activities. Some comments indicated that participants viewed the experience as an opportunity to do or to desire something different. 'I can't live my life as I want to live my life. It's not theirs I want to live [...] it's mine' (TBI 5). Another participant viewed their future in the following manner: 'Well I'd like us to have a more elaborate social life, both for her and for me. To have common passions, leisure activities, to share. But that is up to us. These are things, issues we need to work on' (TBI 2).

Most participants did some thinking about their relationship: 'It did not change anything, but we became more conscious of what it [our relationship] would require' (SO 2). Another participant added 'Ah.., it strengthened our bond [...] It allowed us to spend time together. [...] And to talk to each other a little bit more' (SO 5).

Others reviewed the type of relationship they had with their partner.

> I have always been a protective parent, a parent who initiates everything and who is there to structure my son's entire universe. [...] I am conscious that I am in an over-protective world and in that way, he will not learn and [...] so, I am changing this aspect of my relationship with him and the project was a fine opportunity to try that. Even if it was on the level of communication, it really was about the relationship. (SO 3)

The programme allowed participants to spend quality time together 'And your partner, he's doing something else. And you look at what he's doing and you think, it's a lot of fun' (SO 4). An unexpected benefit revealed by the qualitative results is the fact that the participants enjoyed the discussion times after each meeting, which they used to reflect about their relationships. 'The discussions after each session were more than interesting; it was where relationships were created' (SO 4).

The activities seemed to have been an opportunity for most of the participants to be together differently: 'It really opened my mind and I'm even more convinced that this is a worthwhile cause [...]. That's it, to be, to have a social life, a bit, that helped me' (SO 2). 'I found it interesting, it made us a lot closer, it helped me become a lot closer to my partner' (SO 1).

Through the programme, participants were able to gain a new appreciation of their partner's abilities. SO 1 appreciated the fact that her partner was able to adapt himself, in spite of his own physical limitations, to dance with her and her wheelchair. Another participant (TBI 4) discovered that his partner used to be a very good dancer.

Some participants were attentive to specific aspects of communication, which had changed or were in need of improvement. A participant stated: 'The programme was useful for me, more than for my partner, to assert myself. Yunno get out of my shell, let's say, to assert myself a bit more [...]. As much with her, as with others' (TBI 1). For another participant (SO 2) the improvements reported were that he should become a better listener and to allow his partner to finish his thoughts and really listen to him until the end. Another one (SO 4) recognized that he needed to pay more attention to how he spoke to his partner and to be less emotional, which he thought was difficult to do. Another participant thought that communication was easier with his partner: 'Our time together has changed, we communicate more easily [...] more intimately [...] it's more tempting to communicate to make the move towards him' (TBI3).

In summary, participation in the programme helped both members of the dyad to re-discover one another in a new perspective and revisit their relationship mainly through new experiences acquired within the arts programme. Many participants felt closer, allowing us to believe that the programme has the potential to improve the relationship between partners based on new perceptions of one another and improved communication. 'It's like a communication...you're back in your own land but with new tools...communication tools.... It's like in the language. In fact it's a language in itself' (TBI 3).

Discussion and conclusion

To our knowledge, this is the first study that has investigated the benefits of artistic activities for persons with TBI and a significant other with a focus on interpersonal communication. We recruited five dyads of person with TBI and a significant other interested in communication. All participants reported some benefit from the programme ranging from self-actualization to improvements in their relationships. Although the small number of participants limits the generalizability of the results, these preliminary data are promising and indicate that this programme warrants further study.

A mixed-method design allowed us to examine the impacts of the programme and to complement the few quantitative results with informative qualitative data. Although no differences in communication were measurable statistically, participants were stimulated in thinking about communication and how the programme might be helping them in further exploration of their relationships. It is possible that a reflexive process is the first step necessary for behavioural changes. We must note that participants were neither guided in discussion sessions nor supported in specifically 'doing things' to improve communication or their relationship, which some participants expected, based on previous experience in rehabilitation. Some participants did make changes in their relationship through rediscovering the other and became less situated in the caregiving role and more in a 'normal' relationship with their partner. However, such changes were not picked up with the standardized instruments we had chosen for the study. Both instruments provided a score based on multiple subjective judgements the participants made about themselves and their partner specifically in situations of conversation in their daily life. We should bear in mind that conversation is a more technical aspect of interpersonal communication and relationships, which are both more complex human experiences. Moreover, participants spoke about how the activities in the arts programme were the situations within which changes in perspectives occurred. These changes may be insufficient or take some time to become translated in improved day-to-day conversations. The case could also be made for the minimal insight provided by the standardized instruments for understanding programme effects in comparison with the interviews. The interviews provided a context for the participants to reflect and to make sense of their experience, a process more conducive to introspection than checking numbers on paper. Nevertheless, some participants did report changes in conversations with these instruments, which were lost in the group analyses. A future study will examine more closely the qualitative and quantitative data in a case-by-case manner to describe more accurately which changes may have occurred within each dyad. In future investigations, observational measures of natural conversation between partners may be more informative than the rating scales used in this study.

Some unexpected results also warrant further discussion. Some participants had significantly changed their views in regard to recreational activities shared with their significant other, but in a negative way. It is possible that participants had a more realistic view of what consisted of true pleasant events in their lives outside of the programme after it had ended. In fact, participants were enthusiastic about several of the arts sessions, which had been fun, enjoyable or very interesting.

According to the qualitative analyses, participation in the programme represented a starting point for most of the dyads to improve their relationships through a dynamic adaptive process (Michallet, Tétreault, and Le Dorze 2003). The participants appeared to be more aware of their interactional patterns with their dyad partner and more able to identify means to change and enhance their relationships. However, we had not anticipated such changes, and therefore in subsequent work on this topic appropriate sensitive tools or interview guides are required.

When developing the programme we wanted to create a context where there was no distinction made between care providers and brain-injured care receivers. Using artistic activities with people who had little expertise in the arts allowed everyone to start on the same level and to participate using their own strengths, potential and abilities. Using art experts was another means of ensuring that skilled individuals would lead the activities with experience in teaching arts and in leading groups, therefore improving the chances of success and pleasure for all participants. In fact, our results indicated that participants understood and seized the opportunity to reveal themselves in a new perspective, based on a new awareness of their potential. They discovered that they could do things they did not know about before. No one spoke of his/her experience in terms related to rehabilitation, injury or disability.

During art sessions, participants were placed in situations where they had to pay attention to the different forms of communication required for a specific activity. Sometimes a word, a gesture, an idea, an emotion or a new image took on new meaning, especially through observation. Within this type of context, where creativity and freedom were valued, participants were allowed to focus on the essence of their relationship and on the other person as a potential creator of signs.

According to Fleury, Marazzani, and Saucier (2003), interventions that target the development of very specific abilities may be limited in terms of generalization to other social spheres. However, when the activity stimulates self-esteem and the inner self, generalization is possible. In order for this to occur, both the creative and the playful dimension of the activity need to be tangible. In this regard, a programme such as the one we proposed became an opportunity for facilitating the identity negotiating process, for both the participant and his/her significant other (Lundberg et al. 2011). With these kinds of outcomes, an arts programme does contribute to the social integration of people with TBI as well as their significant other by reducing social isolation (Caldwell 2005).

This study allowed the researchers to analyse the potential of using arts (drawing, theatre and dance) to support interpersonal communication and the relationships between an individual with TBI and his/her significant other. It proposed an innovative approach focused on reinforcing relationships within the dyad through the experience of sharing pleasant moments together. Preliminary data in this small convenience sample are promising and suggest that the intervention could be useful for improving the quality of life of people with TBI, their family members and friends. We also have data that will allow us to choose sensitive ways of measuring and documenting outcomes with an appropriate research design.

Acknowledgements

This study was supported by a research grant awarded to the first two authors as part of an ONF-REPAR (Ontario Neurotrauma Foundation-Réseau de Recherche en Adaptation-Réadaptation du Québec) team grant (2007–2010). We gratefully thank all of our participants for their enthusiastic participation. The participation of the following community associations is acknowledged: Centre d'immersion en arts La Fenêtre et Association des traumatisés crâniens de la Mauricie. We express our thanks to Marie-Christine Hallé et France Bergeron, for their assistance, and to our research assistants: Caroline Mailloux and Laura-Kim Dumesnil.

Notes on contributors

Hélène Carbonneau is a Professor in leisure and health in the department of leisure, culture and tourism studies at Université du Québec à Trois-Rivières, (Canada). She holds a master degree and a PhD in gerontology from Université de Sherbrooke. Her research interests include leisure education, inclusion, gerontology, disabilities and caregiving with a focus on positive aspects and strengths enhancement.

Professor Guylaine Le Dorze is at the School of Speech-Language Therapy and Audiology at the Université de Montréal. She holds a PhD in Linguistics from Université de Montréal. She is a senior researcher at the Centre for Interdisciplinary Research in Rehabilitation of Montreal. Her principal research interests include: communication disorders, aphasia rehabilitation, and psychosocial impacts of communication disorders, families, aging and brain injury.

France Joyal is a professor in art education in the Department of philosophy and arts of the Université du Québec à Trois-Rivières (Canada). Trained in visual arts and dance, she holds a master's degree in arts and a doctorate in education. Her researches concern representation, aesthetic experience, artistic dynamics, cognitive companionship and embodiement. Worried of reducing the ditch between the scientist and pragmatics, she is interested in the methodology of the research in arts and she multiplies the activities of diffusion gathering researchers, professionals and practitioners.

Marie-Josée Plouffe is a professor of theatre in Arts Education in the Department of philosophy and arts of the Université du Québec à Trois-Rivières (Canada). She holds a PhD in Arts and Practices Studies. She is interested by the factors that contribute to learning, enacting/performing and creation.

References

Barth, Britt-Mari. 2002. *Le savoir en construction* [Knowledge in Development]. Paris: Éditions Retz.

Bravo, G., P. Gaulin, and M.-F. Dubois. 1996. "Validation d'une échelle de bien-être général auprès d'une population francophone âgée de 50 à 75 ans [Validation of Well-being Scale with French Speaking Population 50 to 75 Old]." *Canadian Journal on Aging/La Revue canadienne du vieillissement* 15 (1): 112–128. doi:10.1017/S0714980800013325.

Burgoon, J. K., and J. L. Hale. 1987. "Validation and Measurement of the Fundamental Themes of Relational Communication." *Communication Monographs* 54 (1): 19–41. doi:10.1080/03637758709390214.

Caldwell, L. L. 2005. "Leisure and Health: Why is Leisure Therapeutic?" *British Journal of Guidance & Counselling* 33 (1): 7–26. doi:10.1080/03069880412331335939.

Carbonneau, H., É. Martineau, M. Andre, and D. Dawson. 2011. "Enhancing Leisure Experiences Post Traumatic Brain Injury: A Pilot Study." *Brain Impairment* 12 (2): 140–151. doi:10.1375/brim.12.2.140.

Centers for Disease Control and Prevention. 2013. *Get the Stats on Traumatic Brain Injury in the United States*. Traumatic Brain Injury in the United States: Emergency Department Visits, Hospitalizations and Deaths 2002–2006. Atlanta, GA: Department of Health and Human Services. http://www.cdc.gov/traumaticbraininjury/pdf/BlueBook_factsheet-a.pdf.

Corrigan, J. D., J. A. Bogner, W. J. Mysiw, D. Clinchot, and L. Fugate. 2001. "Life Satisfaction after Traumatic Brain Injury." *The Journal of Head Trauma Rehabilitation* 16 (6): 543–555. doi:10.1097/00001199-200112000-00003.

David, I. R. 1999. *An Exploration of the Role of Art as Therapy in Rehabilitation from Traumatic Brain Injury: A Dissertation Submitted*. Cincinnati, OH: Union Institute. http://worldcat.org

Demakis, G. J., F. Hammond, A. Knotts, D. B. Cooper, P. Clement, J. Kennedy, and T. Sawyer. 2007. "The Personality Assessment Inventory in Individuals with Traumatic Brain Injury." *Archives of Clinical Neuropsychology* 22 (1): 123–130. doi:10.1016/j.acn.2006.09.004.

Devine, M. A. 2004. "Being a 'Doer' Instead of a 'Viewer'": The Role of Inclusive Leisure Contexts in Determining Social Acceptance for People with Disabilities." *Journal of Leisure Research* 36 (2): 137–159. http://js.sagamorepub.com/jlr/article/view/569.

Douglas, J. M. 2013. "Conceptualizing Self and Maintaining Social Connection Following Severe Traumatic Brain Injury." *Brain Injury* 27 (1): 60–74. doi:10.3109/02699052.2012.722254.

Douglas, J. M., C. A. O'Flaherty, and P. C. Snow. 2000. "Measuring Perception of Communicative Ability: The Development and Evaluation of the La Trobe Communication Questionnaire." *Aphasiology* 14 (3): 251–268. doi:10.1080/026870300401469.

Driver, B. L., P. J. Brown, and G. L. Peterson. 1991. *Benefits of Leisure*. State College, PA: Venture Publishing.

Dupuy, H. J. 1978. "Self-Representations of General Psychological Well-Being of American Adults." Paper presented at American Public Health Association Meeting, Los Angeles, California, October 17.

Fleury, F., M. H. Marazzani, and J.-F. Saucier. 2003. "Le jeu théâtral comme inducteur de changement dans les habiletés sociales [Drama Play as Change Inductor of Social Skills]." *Santé mentale au Québec* 28 (2): 251–272. doi:10.7202/008627ar.

Foster, A. M., J. Armstrong, A. Buckley, J. Sherry, T. Young, S. Foliaki, and K. M. McPherson. 2012. "Encouraging Family Engagement in the Rehabilitation Process: A Rehabilitation Provider's Development of Support Strategies for Family Members of People with Traumatic Brain Injury." *Disability and Rehabilitation* 34 (22): 1855–1862. doi:10.3109/09638288.2012.670028.

Goodman, N. 1968. *Languages of Art: An Approach to A Theory of Symbols*. Indianapolis: Bobbs-Merril.

Goodman, N. 1992. *Manières de faire des mondes* [Ways to Do World]. Paris: Gallimard.

Hale, J. L., J. K. Burgoon, and B. Householder. 2005. "The Relational Communication Scale." In *The Sourcebook of Nonverbal Measures: Going Beyond Words*, edited by V. Manusov, 119–132. Mahwah, NJ: Lawrence Erlbaum.

Hutchinson, S. L., D. P. Loy, D. A. Kleiber, and J. Dattilo. 2003. "Leisure as a Coping Resource: Variations in Coping with Traumatic Injury and Illness." *Leisure Sciences* 25 (2–3): 143–161. doi:10.1080/01490400306566.

Institut National en Santé Publique du Québec. 2012. *Évolution des hospitalisations attribuables aux traumatismes craniocérébraux d'origine non intentionnelle au Québec* [Hospitalisation Evolution Relate to Non-intentional Traumatic Brain Injury in Québec]. Quebec: Ministère de l'Éducation, du Loisir et du Sport du Québec.

Iwasaki, Y., J. MacTavish, and K. MacKay. 2005. "Building on Strengths and Resilience: Leisure as a Stress Survival Strategy." *British Journal of Guidance & Counselling* 33 (1): 81–100. doi:10.1080/03069880412331335894.

Kagan, A., S. E. Black, J. F. Duchan, N. Simmons-Mackie, and P. Square. 2001. "Training Volunteers as Conversation Partners Using 'Supported Conversation for Adults With Aphasia' (SCA): A Controlled Trial." *Journal of Speech Language and Hearing Research* 44 (3): 624–638. doi:10.1044/1092-4388(2001/051).

Lammel, J. A. 2003. "Relationship between Dimensions of Leisure Activity Experience, Sense of Coherence, and Psychological Well-Being for Traumatic Brain Injury Survivors." PhD diss., The Pennsylvania State University.

Leclerc, G., L. Montminy, and C. Noiseux. 1989. *Un instrument multifonctionnel de mesure d'attitudes: Ministère de l'enseignement supérieur et de la science* [Multifunctional Attitudes Measurement Tool]. Direction générale de l'enseignement collégial.

Le Dorze, G., and C. Brassard. 1995. "A Description of the Consequences of Aphasia on Aphasic Persons and Their Relatives and Friends, Based on the WHO Model of Chronic Diseases." *Aphasiology* 9 (3): 239–255. doi:10.1080/02687039508248198.

Lefebvre, H., G. Cloutier, and M. J. Levert. 2008. "Perspectives of Survivors of Traumatic Brain Injury and Their Caregivers on Long-Term Social Integration." *Brain Injury* 22(7–8): 535–543. doi:10.1080/02699050802158243.

Lefebvre, H., Désilets, M., & Ndakengurukiye, G. 2004. *La participation sociale à long terme des personnes ayant subi un traumatisme crânien et l'impact chez les proches, 10 ans post-traumatisme* [Long Term Social Participation of People with Traumatic Brain Injury and Impact for Significant Others 10 Years Post-trauma]. Translated by F. D. S. infirmières. Montréal: Université de Montréal.

LoBello, S. G., A. T. Underhil, P. V. Valentine, T. P. Stroud, A. A. Bartolucci, and P. R. Fine. 2003. "Social Integration and Life and Family Satisfaction in Survivors of Injury at 5 Years Post Injury." *Journal of Rehabilitation Research and Development* 40 (4): 293–300. http://www.rehab.research.va.gov/jour/03/40/4/lobello.html.

Lomas, J., L. Pickard, S. Bester, H. Elbard, A. Finlayson, and C. Zoghaib. 1989. "The Communicative Effectiveness Index: Development and Psychometric Evaluation of a Functional Communication Measure for Adult Aphasia." *Journal of Speech Language and Hearing Research* 54 (1): 113–124. http://jshd.asha.org/cgi/content/abstract/54/1/113.

Lundberg, N. R., S. Taniguchi, B. P. McCormick, and C. Tibbs. 2011. "Identity Negotiating: Redefining Stigmatized Identities through Adaptive Sports and Recreation Participation among Individuals with a Disability." *Journal of Leisure Research* 43 (2): 5–225.

McDonald, S. 2013. "Impairments in Social Cognition Following Severe Traumatic Brain Injury." *Journal of the International Neuropsychological Society* 19 (3): 231–246. doi:10.1017/S1355617712001506.

Michallet, B., S. Tétreault, and G. Le Dorze. 2003. "The Consequences of Severe Aphasia on the Spouses of Aphasic People: A Description of the Adaptation Process." *Aphasiology* 17 (9): 835–859. doi:10.1080/02687030344000238.

Paillé, P., and A. Mucchielli. 2012. *L'analyse qualitative en sciences humaines et sociales* [Qualitative Analysis in Human and Social Sciences]. Paris: Armand Colin.

Perlesz, A., G. Kinsella, and S. Crowe. 2000. "Psychological Distress and Family Satisfaction Following Traumatic Brain Injury: Injured Individuals and Their Primary, Secondary, and

Tertiary Carers." *Journal of Head Trauma Rehabilitation* 15 (3): 909–929. doi:10.1097/00001199-200006000-00005.

Reynolds, F. 2003. "Exploring the Meanings of Artistic Occupation for Women Living with Chronic Illness: A Comparison of Template and Interpretative Phenomenological Approaches to Analysis." *The British Journal of Occupational Therapy* 66 (12): 551–558. http://www.ingentaconnect.com/content/cot/bjot/2003/00000066/00000012/art00003.

Reynolds, F., B. Vivat, and S. Prior. 2008. "Women's Experiences of Increasing Subjective Well-Being in CFS/ME Through Leisure-Based Arts and Crafts Activities: A Qualitative Study." *Disability and Rehabilitation* 30 (17): 1279–1288. doi:10.1080/09638280701654518.

Rhondali, W., M. Barmaki, A. Laurent, and M. Filbet. 2007. "L'art jusqu'au bout de la vie [Art Until the End of Life]." *Psycho-Oncologie* 1 (3): 195–199. doi:10.1007/s11839-007-0031-3.

Rietdijk, R., L. Togher, and E. Power. 2012. "Supporting Family Members of People with Traumatic Brain Injury Using Telehealth: A Systematic Review." *Journal of Rehabilitation Medicine* 44 (11): 913–921. doi:10.1007/s11839-007-1058.

Salois-Bellerose, E., C. Croteau, and G. Le Dorze. 2008. *Une adaptation du Relational Communication Scale pour l'évaluation de la communication de couples touchés par l'aphasie* [Adaptation of Relational Communication Scale for Communicaion Evaluation of Couples Effected by Aphasia]. Rapport de stage de recherche. Université de Montréal.

Siegel, S., and N. J. Castellan. 1988. *Nonparametric Statistics for the Behavioral Sciences*. 2nd ed. New-York: McGraw-Hill.

Steadman-Pare, D., A. Colantonio, G. Ratcliff, S. Chase, and L. Vernich. 2001. "Factors Associated with Perceived Quality of Life Many Years after Traumatic Brain Injury." *The Journal of Head Trauma Rehabilitation* 16 (4): 330–342. doi:10.1097/00001199-200108000-00004.

Stern, Daniel N. 2004. *The Present Moment in Psychotherapy and Everyday Life*. New York: W.W. Norton.

Turner, B., J. Fleming, J. Parry, M. Vromans, P. Cornwell, C. Gordon, and T. Ownsworth. 2010. "Caregivers of Adults with Traumatic Brain Injury: The Emotional Impact of Transition from Hospital to Home." *Brain Impairment* 11 (3): 281–292. doi:10.1375/brim.11.3.281.

Ylvisaker, M., L. S. Turkstra, and C. Coelho. 2005. "Behavioral and Social Interventions for Individuals with Traumatic Brain Injury: A Summary of the Research with Clinical Implications." *Seminars in Speech and Language* 26 (4): 256–267. doi:10.1055/s-2005-922104.

Zumbo, B. D. 2003. "Leisure Activities, Health and Quality of Life." In *Essays on the Quality of Life*, edited by A. Michalos, Vol. 19, 217–238. Netherlands: Kluwer Academic Publishers.

Index

Note: Page numbers in **bold** type refer to figures
Page numbers in *italic* type refer to tables

DATE DUE	RETURNED